# Ovid on Cosmetics

Also available from Bloomsbury

*Ovid and his Love Poetry*, Rebecca Armstrong
*The Metamorphosis of Ovid*, Sarah Annes Brown
*Prescribing Ovid*, Yasmin Haskell
*Ovid's Myth of Pygmalion on Screen*, Paula James
*Ovid's 'Metamorphoses'*, Genevieve Liveley
*Ovid: Love Songs*, Genevieve Liveley

# Ovid on Cosmetics

*Medicamina Faciei Femineae* and Related Texts

Marguerite Johnson

Bloomsbury Academic
An imprint of Bloomsbury Publishing Plc

B L O O M S B U R Y
LONDON • OXFORD • NEW YORK • NEW DELHI • SYDNEY

**Bloomsbury Academic**
An imprint of Bloomsbury Publishing Plc

50 Bedford Square   1385 Broadway
London              New York
WC1B 3DP            NY 10018
UK                  USA

www.bloomsbury.com

**BLOOMSBURY and the Diana logo are trademarks of Bloomsbury Publishing Plc**

First published 2016

© Marguerite Johnson, 2016

Marguerite Johnson has asserted her right under the Copyright, Designs and Patents Act, 1988, to be identified as Author of this work.

All rights reserved. No part of this publication may be reproduced or transmitted in any form or by any means, electronic or mechanical, including photocopying, recording, or any information storage or retrieval system, without prior permission in writing from the publishers.

No responsibility for loss caused to any individual or organization acting on or refraining from action as a result of the material in this publication can be accepted by Bloomsbury or the author.

**British Library Cataloguing-in-Publication Data**
A catalogue record for this book is available from the British Library.

ISBN:  HB:    978-1-47251-442-4
       PB:    978-1-47250-657-3
       ePDF:  978-1-47250-674-0
       ePub:  978-1-47250-749-5

**Library of Congress Cataloging-in-Publication Data**
Ovid, 43 B.C–17 A.D. or 18 A.D.
Ovid on cosmetics : Medicamina faciei femineae and related texts /
[Ovid] ; Marguerite Johnson.
pages cm
Includes bibliographical references and index.
ISBN 978-1-4725-1442-4 (hardback) — ISBN 978-1-4725-0657-3 (pb) —
ISBN 978-1-4725-0749-5 (epub)   1. Cosmetics—Poetry—Early works to 1800.
2. Didactic poetry, Latin—Translations into English.   3. Ovid, 43 B.C.–17 A.D. or
18 A.D.—Criticism and interpretation.   I. Johnson, Marguerite, 1965– author, translator.
II. Ovid, 43 B.C–17 A.D. or 18 A.D. De medicamine faciei.   III. Ovid, 43 B.C–17 A.D.
or 18 A.D. De medicamine faciei. English.   IV. Ovid, 43 B.C.–17 A.D. or
18 A.D. Ars Amatoria. Selections.   V. Ovid, 43 B.C–17 A.D. or 18 A.D. Ars Amatoria.
Selections. English.   VI. Ovid, 43 B.C.–17 A.D. or 18 A.D. Amores. Selections.
VII. Ovid, 43 B.C.–17 A.D. or 18 A.D. Amores. Selections. English.
VIII. Title. PA6519.D4O95 2015
871'.01–dc23
2015018895

Typeset by RefineCatch Limited, Bungay, Suffolk

*To my daughter, Katherine Scarlett Beatrix Johnson,
whose face gleams like golden flowers.*

# Contents

| | |
|---|---|
| List of Illustrations | viii |
| Preface | x |
| Acknowledgements | xii |
| Ovid's Works | xiii |
| Introduction | 1 |
| 1   *Medicamina Faciei Femineae* | 41 |
| 2   *Amores* 1.14 | 83 |
| 3   *Ars Amatoria* 3.101–250 | 97 |
| 4   *Remedia Amoris* 343–356 | 125 |
| 5   *Ars Amatoria* 1.505–524 | 131 |
| Appendices | 137 |
| Appendix 1: Notes on the Latin texts | 137 |
| Appendix 2: Glossary of cosmeceutical terminology | 141 |
| Appendix 3: Ingredients in the *Medicamina* recipes | 142 |
| Appendix 4: Roman weights and measures and equivalents | 142 |
| Bibliography | 143 |
| Index of Passages | 159 |
| General Index | 167 |

# Illustrations

1. Roman container with cosmeceutical cream. Mid-second century AD. © Museum of London. — 11
2. Bronze cosmetics container. Fourth to third century BC. The Metropolitan Museum of Art/Art Resource. © Photo SCALA, Florence. — 12
3. Box containing toiletries, from Cumae, Campania. First century AD. National Archaeological Museum, Naples. © Photo SCALA, Florence. — 13
4. Gilded bronze mirror depicting the Three Graces. Second century AD. The Metropolitan Museum of Art/Art Resource. © Photo SCALA, Florence. — 14
5. Roman double-sided ivory comb. First century BC to second century AD. © Johns Hopkins Archaeological Museum. — 14
6. Stele of P. Ferrarius Hermes. First century BC to second century AD. © Museo della Civiltà Romana. — 15
7. Barley (*Hordeum vulgare*). Robert Bentley. *Medicinal plants*... (London: J. & A. Churchill, 1875–1880). Vol. 4. Plate 293. Courtesy Royal Botanic Gardens, Kew. — 62
8. Bitter vetch (*Ervum ervilia* [sic]). Joseph Jacob Ritter von Plenck. *Icones plantarum medicinalium*... (Viennae: Apud Rudolphum Graeffer et Soc., 1788–1812). Vol. 6. Plate 566. Courtesy Royal Botanic Gardens, Kew. — 63
9. Narcissus (*Flora Parisiensis*). Pierre Bulliard (Paris: P. Fr. Didot le Jeune, Libraire, quai des Augustins, 1776–1783). Vol. 2. Plate 170. Courtesy Royal Botanic Gardens, Kew. — 66
10. White lupin (*Lupinus albus*). Johannes Zorn. *Icones plantarum medicinalium* (Nürnberg: auf Kosten der Raspischen Buchhandlung, 1779–1790). Vol. 4. Plate 321. Courtesy Royal Botanic Gardens, Kew. — 69

11. Fennel (*Foeniculum vulgare*). James Sowerby. *English botany, or, Coloured figures of British plants* (London: Hardwicke, 1863–1886). Vol. 4. Plate 601. Courtesy Royal Botanic Gardens, Kew.     79

# Preface

This book is about Ovid's interest in female beautification with an emphasis on cosmetics and cosmeceuticals, the related accoutrements of clothing and jewellery, and the knowledge, technology and science that underlie them. As such it privileges the somewhat neglected *Medicamina Faciei Femineae* (*Treatments for the Female Face*). It also extends its textual reach to *Amores* 1.14, a section from *Ars Amatoria* Book Three, and a passage each from *Remedia Amoris* and *Ars Amatoria* Book One (on male adornment). Ultimately, what becomes clear is not only the breadth and depth of Ovid's knowledge of the arcana of the *mundus muliebris* ('woman's toilette') but that of its owners as well.

In addition to the technical knowledge contained in the *Medicamina* and the related passages, the works reveal Roman attitudes towards cosmetics and cosmeceuticals and Ovid's opinions on them. This book also addresses such opinions, juxtaposing Ovid's views to those of his predecessors and contemporaries to underscore the contested history of female adornment in Rome. As such it considers attendant themes such as the value system Ovid applies to adornment, namely *cultus*, *mollitia* and *ars*, and explores the links between the embellished female body, sexualities and moralities. In this respect the study follows Ovid's cues as it engages with a complex mix of beauty products, hair treatments, jewellery and fine clothes, entangled with issues pertaining to female agency at a crucial time in the history of Roman women. As women of the early imperial age attempted to participate in the material opportunities proffered by national prosperity and international trade, they encountered a new state authority with a moral agenda that aimed to take both them, and their male guardians, back to a pristine, idealized past. Ovid is the self-appointed chronicler of all these interrelated and competing dialogues, capturing a significant moment in time while simultaneously injecting his works with a suite of poetic techniques, which also require attention.

In view of all this, the book, like much of Ovid's work, retains a hybridity, as it constantly attempts to harness (almost) too many things at once. With cosmetics and cosmeceuticals as its focus, it may be best described as a cultural-literary analysis and, therefore, not limited to a specific audience. Instead it aims to make a modest contribution to the post-postmodern shift in the direction of a shedding of the rigidities of scholarly disciplines and specified scholarship within them, offering instead some useful information to divergent lines of enquiry.

A new translation of the *Medicamina* and the related passages are provided with a focus on accuracy rather than artistic interpretation on the translator's part. Each translation is accompanied by a Latin text based on Kenney's 1995 edition with significant textual variations or problems noted in Appendix 1. While it is anticipated that many readers will be interested in the contents of the poems rather than the Latinity, the Latin text and notes have been provided for those who prefer to read the passages in the original. As the text is not aimed at undergraduate language students, grammatical points and related apparati have not been included (although the details provided on the individual ingredients listed, particularly in the *Medicamina*, may prove useful to Latin classes studying the passages).

The Commentaries are usually structured according to the sequential unfolding of themes in each piece and, only occasionally, on individual couplets. Accordingly, headings are used to highlight section topics. While this approach is somewhat artificial, it reinforces the structure of each poem or excerpt and, for the purpose of clarity of analysis, is an effective means of dealing with the, at times, overabundance of information in the first three texts. The four passages that follow the *Medicamina* each have a brief introduction at the start of the Commentaries in order to provide a poetic context for them. In view of the comparatively small length of passages four and five, *Remedia Amoris* 343–356 and *Ars Amatoria* 1.505–524, these Commentaries take the form of small essays.

For readability, abbreviations have been kept to a minimum in the Commentaries and have been applied only to titles by Ovid. Several authors have been consistently cited and are referenced by name and textual section only; these authors and texts are: Celsus, *On Medicine*; Dioscorides, *On Medical Substances*; and Pliny the Elder, *Natural History*. All other ancient authors and texts are cited in full.

# Acknowledgements

I would like to thank Terry Ryan for sharing his versions of the texts, working with me on the *Medicamina* translation and discussing the Latin variants in the manuscripts. Terry also provided the photograph for the cover. While writing the book, I received invaluable advice from John Scarborough on various cosmeceutical ingredients, Barbara Weiden Boyd on *Amores* 1.14 and Tim Leary on passages from the *Medicamina*. Kymme Laetsch provided superb research assistance. Thomas Sharkie was an excellent proofreader. Alice Wright and Anna MacDiarmid from Bloomsbury were consistently helpful, particularly in relation to organizing the images, and selecting two excellent anonymous readers who provided wise advice. When the manuscript came close to a penultimate draft, Lindsay and Patricia Watson read it in its entirety, providing numerous suggestions and corrections for which I am incredibly grateful; this book is so much better for their astute comments. Finally, thank you to Leni, Jack and Kate for their love, support and patience.

# Ovid's Works

| Dates     | Works                      | Abbreviations |
|-----------|----------------------------|---------------|
| 19 BC     | *Heroides* 1–15 (?)        | *Her.*        |
| 16–15 BC  | *Amores* (1st ed.)         | *Am.*         |
| 8–3 BC    | *Amores* (2nd ed.)         | *Am.*         |
| 2 BC      | *Medicamina Faciei Femineae* | *Med.*      |
| 2 BC      | *Ars Amatoria* (1 and 2)   | *AA / Ars*    |
| AD 2      | *Ars Amatoria* (3)         | *AA / Ars*    |
| AD 2      | *Remedia Amoris*           | *Rem.*        |
| AD 3–7    | *Fasti*                    | *Fast.*       |
| AD 3–8    | *Metamorphoses*            | *Met.*        |
| AD 9–12   | *Tristia* (1–5)            | *Tr.*         |
| AD 13     | *Epistles* (1–3)           | *Ep.*         |
| AD 14–16  | *Epistles* (4)             | *Ep.*         |

# Introduction

## Now and then ... making-over a woman

It is fascinating to hypothesize Ovid's views on the cosmeceutical and cosmetic industry in the modern west. Equally intriguing would be his opinion on elective cosmetic surgery. Both industries, driven by increasingly high consumer demand, have yearly profits in the billions of pounds as women, and increasingly men, seek to improve, preserve and even alter their appearance. Each year millions of women undergo procedures such as Botox injections, chemical peels, liposuctions, breast augmentations or reductions, laser hair removal, even calf augmentation and vaginal rejuvenation surgery. Research has estimated that cosmetic surgery in the United States will increase from approximately 1,688,694 patients in 2012, to 3,847,929 in 2030 with more and more men contributing to this projected figure (Broer, Levine and Juran 2014).

The strangeness inherent in an ancient Roman's hypothetical encounter with modern beautification, as fanciful as the thought may be, underlines the implicit wonderment and anxiety-inducing responses that characterize the phenomenon. Transforming women into goddesses and men into gods through artificial means would surely have struck people from antiquity as somewhat miraculous in terms of surgical virtuosity but also perhaps as an ill-omened procedure that unwisely erased the physical demarcations between divinity and mortal. This is not to suggest, however, that the Romans were unfamiliar with plastic surgery. Celsus (7.8) records otoplasty to repair damage to the ears caused by heavy earrings (cf. Barini 1958: 43), procedures to repair parts of the body from the nose (Celsus: 7.10) to the mouth (7.12), and surgery to restore the prepuce (posthioplasty) for an aesthetically pleasing appendage (cf. Hodges 2001).

Even the application of a simple 'patch' (*aluta*), to which Ovid refers at *AA* 3.202, indicates awareness of body modification for the purpose of a more appealing exterior. These leather patches concealed unsightly blemishes and were also used to hide tattoos on the bodies of manumitted slaves (cf. Jones 1987). Martial, who refers to the doctors skilled in the removal of slave tattoos at 6.64.26 and 10.56.6, also mentions patches at 2.29.9–10 and 8.33.22 (where they are called *splenia*). In an age in which cosmetic technologies were comparatively rudimentary, patches were one of the few options available for improving one's appearance, but if laser treatment had been invented, surely the Romans would have taken advantage of it.

Such fantasies and hypotheses may not seem so far-fetched when one considers a fragment from the *Isostasion* or *The Equivalent*, a play by the Alexandrian comedian, Alexis (*The Fragments*: 103 Arnott 1996), and recorded by Athenaeus (568a–d). The passage discusses courtesans and the procuress's modification of their bodies to meet clients' individual tastes:

πρῶτα μὲν γὰρ πρὸς τὸ κέρδος καὶ τὸ συλᾶν τοὺς πέλας
πάντα τἄλλ' αὐταῖς πάρεργα γίνεται, ῥάπτουσι δὲ
πᾶσιν ἐπιβουλάς. ἐπειδὰν δ' εὐπορήσωσίν ποτε,
ἀνέλαβον καινὰς ἑταίρας, πρωτοπείρους τῆς τέχνης·
εὐθὺς ἀναπλάττουσι ταύτας, ὥστε μήτε τοὺς τρόπους
μήτε τὰς ὄψεις ὁμοίας διατελεῖν οὔσας ἔτι.
τυγχάνει μικρά τις οὖσα· φελλὸς ἐν ταῖς βαυκίσιν      b
ἐγκεκάττυται. μακρά τις· διάβαθρον λεπτὸν φορεῖ
τήν τε κεφαλὴν ἐπὶ τὸν ὦμον καταβαλοῦσ' ἐξέρχεται·
τοῦτο τοῦ μήκους ἀφεῖλεν. οὐκ ἔχει τις ἰσχία·
ὑπενέδυσ' ἐρραμέν' αὐτήν, ὥστε τὴν εὐπυγίαν
ἀναβοᾶν τοὺς εἰσιδόντας. κοιλίαν ἁδρὰν ἔχει·
στηθί' ἔστ' αὐταῖσι τούτων ὧν ἔχουσ' οἱ κωμικοί·
ὀρθὰ προσθεῖσαι τοιαῦτα τοὔκλυτον τῆς κοιλίας
ὡσπερεὶ κοντοῖσι τούτοις εἰς τὸ πρόσθ' ἀπήγαγον.     c
τὰς ὀφρῦς πυρρὰς ἔχει τις· ζωγραφοῦσιν ἀσβόλῳ.
συμβέβηκ' εἶναι μέλαιναν· κατέπλασεν ψιμυθίῳ.
λευκόχρως λίαν τίς ἐστιν· παιδέρωτ' ἐντρίβεται.
καλὸν ἔχει τοῦ σώματός τι· τοῦτο γυμνὸν δείκνυται.
εὐφυεῖς ὀδόντας ἔσχεν· ἐξ ἀνάγκης δεῖ γελᾶν,
ἵνα θεωρῶσ' οἱ παρόντες τὸ στόμ' ὡς κομψὸν φορεῖ.

ἂν δὲ μὴ χαίρῃ γελῶσα, διατελεῖ τὴν ἡμέραν  d
ἔνδον, ὥσπερ τοῖς μαγείροις ἃ παράκειθ' ἑκάστοτε,
ἡνίκ' ἂν πωλῶσιν αἰγῶν κρανία, ξυλήφιον
μυρρίνης ἔχουσα λεπτὸν ὀρθὸν ἐν τοῖς χείλεσιν·
ὥστε τῷ χρόνῳ σέσηρεν, ἄν τε βούλητ' ἄν τε μή.
[ὄψεις διὰ τούτων σκευοποιοῦσι τῶν τεχνῶν.]

First, for gain and to swindle their male neighbours,
all other things become secondary to them, but they weave
plots against all men. When at some time they become rich
they take new courtesans who are making their first experiments in the trade.
At once they remake these girls, so that neither their behaviour
nor their appearance remains the same any more.
One girl happens to be little: cork is stitched to the sole of her  b
ladies' shoes. One girl happens to be tall: she wears a thin slipper,
and she goes out drooping her head on her shoulders, which
takes away some of her height. One girl doesn't have a derrière:
she dresses her with sewn-on haunches, under her clothes are stitched hips,
so that those who see her cry out that she has beautiful buttocks.
She has a bulky stomach: for such ones they have false bosoms
made of the materials that the comedy actors have.
After adding these and setting them straight like props,
they bring the clothing away from the belly in front.  c
One girl has red eyebrows: they paint them with soot.
One girl happens to be black: she plasters her with white lead.
One girl is too pale: she rubs on rouge.
She has one part of the body beautiful: she shows it naked.
She has pretty teeth: she must, of necessity, smile so that
the men present may see what an elegant mouth she has.
But if she does not enjoy smiling, she spends the day  d
indoors and, like things displayed by butchers
when they sell goats' heads,
holding upright between her teeth, a thin stick of myrtle;
so that in time she shows her teeth whether she likes it or not.
[By these crafts they artfully prepare their appearance.]

This passage reflects the application of cosmetics such as lead foundation and rouge, as well as more intrusive interventions to modify the body such as false haunches and bosoms and the insertion of a myrtle stick in the mouth to force a smile that reveals teeth. A passage such as this, which may have influenced *AA*.3.255–286 on compensation for natural flaws, and *Rem*. 325–342 on accentuating flaws as a cure for passion, indicates that the ancients interpreted the female body as adaptable or open to transformation, and made an association between female beauty and artificial adornment. Perhaps then, the modern obsession with the quest for youthful beauty, manifest in cosmeceuticals, cosmetics and plastic surgery, may be the end result of an evolutionary trajectory from before the time of Ovid.[1]

Of course, like today's opponents of body modification, there were ancient critics of female beautification procedures. The passage from the *Isostasion* refers to the alteration of the bodies of the courtesans as *technē*, a 'skill' or 'art', but also a deception or sleight of hand. *technē* is essentially the same as the Latin word *ars*; a term employed by Ovid, particularly on beauty and beautification, but not usually with negative connotations. That Ovid does not usually judge feminine *ars* harshly is in contrast to other ancient sources. In Xenophon's *Oeconomicus* (10.2–9), for example, Ischomachus provides an anecdote about teaching his wife to heed his philosophical warnings about dressing-up. Observing her wearing too much make-up and high-heels, Ischomachus asks her whether she would prefer him to deceive her with untruthful tales of exaggerated wealth, showering her with fake luxuries. Of course, his wife replies in the negative. Next he asks her if she would like him to apply rouge and smear foundation under his eyes, then seek her embrace like a cheating consort presenting himself to his mistress. Again, she replies in the negative. The questions and answers inevitably lead Ischomachus's wife to realize the implicitly deceptive and artificial nature of cosmetics.[2]

Xenophon's *Oeconomicus* is a Socratic dialogue, an instructional prose treatise on agriculture and the management of one's house. Its endorsement of a morally upright life naturally caters for a section such as the one on cosmetics. The anti-cosmetic tradition, however, is also expressed in many other genres, including comedy, elegy and satire. In *The Haunted House*, for example, Plautus's character, Scapha ridicules cosmetics (*ll*.258–264) and perfumes (*ll*.273–278), exclaiming at *l*.273: *mulier recte olet, ubi nihil olet* ('a woman smells right, when she smells of nothing'). Scapha believes that young women should let their natural beauty shine without embellishment, while old women who resort to artificial treatments are nothing short of hideous (*ll*.274–277):

> Nam istae veteres, quae se unguentis unctitant, interpoles,
> vetulae, edentulae, quae vitia corporis fuco occulunt,
> ubi sese sudor cum unguentis consociavit, ilico
> itidem olent, quasi cum una multa iura confudit cocus.

> Now those old women, who besmear themselves with ointments, refurbished,
> elderly, toothless, who hide the blemishes of the body with paint,
> when their sweat mixes with ointments, immediately
> they stink, as when a cook mixes many sauces together.

Of course, like Alexis's *Isostasion*, this is comedy. Nevertheless it reflects a common, albeit exaggerated, response to cosmetics. Some 250 years after Plautus, Seneca the Younger in a letter to his mother, *To Helvia, on Consolation* (16), praises her for never having defiled (*polluere*) her face (*facies*) with tints (*colores*) and meretricious adornment (*lenocinium*). Elsewhere, in one of his moral essays, *On Benefits* (7.9), he passes severe judgement on women who wear extravagant garments and jewellery:

> Video uniones non singulos singulis auribus comparatos; iam enim exercitatae aures oneri ferundo sunt; iunguntur inter se et insuper alii binis superponuntur. Non satis muliebris insania viros superiecerat, nisi bina ac terna patrimonia auribus singulis pependissent. Video sericas vestes, si vestes vocandae sunt, in quibus nihil est, quo defendi aut corpus aut denique pudor possit, quibus sumptis parum liquido nudam se non esse iurabit. Hae ingenti summa ab ignotis etiam ad commercium gentibus accersuntur, ut matronae nostrae ne adulteris quidem plus sui in cubiculo, quam in publico ostendant.

> I see this cluster of pearls, not single pearls attached to each ear, because these days ears must be able to carry a weight; the pearls are joined to each other and others are placed on top of the pairs. This womanly insanity had not sufficiently transcended men, unless they hung two or three inheritances from each ear. I see silk dresses, if they can be called dresses, in which there is nothing to protect the body or for that matter a sense of modesty, which,

upon donning, she will scarcely be able to claim unequivocally that she isn't naked. These are fetched at a great price from regions unknown even to trade in order that our matrons may not show more of themselves to their lovers in their bedrooms than they do in public.

Criticism of female luxury, adornment and use of cosmetics is also found between the ages of Plautus (254–184 BC) and Seneca (4 BC–AD 65), throughout the age of Plutarch (AD 45–120) and into the Christian era, providing a consistent tradition of attitudes, be they exaggerated, comic or moral. Poets closer to Ovid's era, Lucretius (99–55 BC) and Horace (65–8 BC) also express anti-adornment views. In the didactic work, *On the Nature of Things* (4.1121–1191), Lucretius warns against the dangers of passion, emphasizing that it blinds men to the covetous and vain nature of women who demand luxury items, including imported perfumes, clothing and jewellery. Horace, in *Satire* 1.2.123–124, claims adornment should be in keeping with nature and, in *Epode* 12.10–11, he furnishes a mocking image of a woman's melting make-up. The natural historian, Pliny the Elder (23–79 AD), writing roughly contemporaneously with Seneca and Plutarch, includes some sneers, such as the one at women wearing pearls on their feet and sandals (9.114). Pliny (13.20–25) also dislikes perfume, associating it with adulterous women and regarding it as the epitome of waste; expensive and prone to evaporation, it is even more decadent than pearls (which can at least be bequeathed). Satirists Martial (AD 40–102) and Juvenal (d. *c.* AD 130) provide various negative tropes associated with beautification (cf. Martial 2.41.11–12 on runny make-up and Juvenal 6.457–507 on the moral turpitude associated with female adornment, including cosmetics).[3]

The Roman elegists also expressed anxieties about, and dislike of, feminine adornment. Propertius (*c.* 50–15 BC), for example, is unimpressed by artificial enhancements:

1.2.7–8:

Crede mihi, non ulla tuae est medicina figurae:
   nudus Amor formae non amat artificem.

Believe me, no doctoring [*medicina*] is needed for your form [*figura*]:
   naked Amor does not love the artificial creator [*artifex*] of beauty [*forma*].

2.18.23–28:

Nunc etiam infectos demens imitare Britannos,
    ludis et externo tincta nitore caput?
Ut natura dedit, sic omnis recta figura est:
    turpis Romano Belgicus ore color.
Illi sub terris fiant mala multa puellae,                                           5
    quae mentita suas vertit inepta comas

Oh mad one, do you now even imitate the dyed [*infectos*] Britons,
    and play the coquette with a foreign tint [*nitor*] on a dyed [*tincta*] head?
Looks as nature bestowed them are always most becoming;
    Belgian colour on a Roman face is ugly.
Let many evils come to that girl in the underworld,                     5
    who in her stupidity cheated and altered her tresses.

Ovid makes similar statements in *Ars* Book Three and *Remedia*, although there is a different rhetorical context for each criticism. In *AA* 3.211–218 he categorically states that applying cosmeceuticals in front of a lover is unadvisable because it looks unattractive and the smell of lanolin is awful. In *Rem.* 351–356 he advises any man who wants to get over a lover to witness her at her toilette (not a pretty sight).

    The anti-cosmetic tradition has several motifs used as justification for an author's opinion. Cosmetics as well as ornate hair and clothing conceal facets of the real woman and are thus essentially deceitful. Additionally, they are artificial and thus not only contradict genuine feminine beauty but attempt to defy the laws of nature. Such accoutrements are also antithetical to perceived notions – particularly vocal in the Augustan age – of the ancestral traditions of Rome, which symbolized simplicity, modesty and chastity. They are consistently associated with the *meretrix* ('courtesan') or adulterous wife as evidenced in the passages above. As symptomatic of stereotypical feminine covetousness they also placed unnecessary financial burdens on men. Barton (2002: 221–222) considers such arguments within the context of *pudicitia* ('chastity') or, more specifically, its antonym, *impudicitia* ('immodesty'): 'Wearing *obvious* make-up ... proclaimed one's unwillingness to be ashamed ... Hiding behind painted-on blush proclaimed not one's blushing modesty but one's brazen shamelessness'.[4] Finally, cosmetics are prone to instability – they melt, 'run' and smear – and thus achieve the opposite result of their intended purpose. Juvenal (6.463) presents a comically exaggerated picture of the mucky nature of lotions in the image of a husband virtually glued to his wife's face when he attempts to kiss her.

## High maintenance ... the Roman body

Despite condemnation, cosmetics have an extensive history throughout the ancient Mediterranean. Like today, there was a distinction between cosmeceuticals and cosmetics in antiquity. Galen (12.434–435, 445–446, 449–450 Kühn 1826), writing in the second century AD, notes the difference between *kosmētikon* ('cosmeceutical') and *kommōtikon* ('cosmetic'). A cosmeceutical designed to enhance the skin by means of, for example, moisturizing it, was acceptable. But the application of a cosmetic such as rouge or skin whitener was deemed inappropriate, unsightly and even immoral. Similarly, applying a medicant to stimulate hair growth or to alleviate dandruff was something standard for both men and women, but dyeing one's hair was regarded as garish, unnecessary and subject to opprobrium. Galen disliked any form of *kommōtikon* but endorsed the use of *kosmētikon* to treat medical conditions such as alopecia (12.432–435 Kühn 1826). Typical of ancient medical texts, Galen's works reference other authors' treatments. He cites recipes preserved in the work entitled *Kosmētikon*, written by Cleopatra (*fl.* first century BC / first century AD),[5] including a hair treatment that consisted of burnt mice, burnt wine dregs, burnt horse teeth, bear fat, deer marrow and reed bark mixed with honey (12.404 Kühn 1826). In addition to Cleopatra, Galen cites other authors of both cosmeceutical and cosmetic treatises, including Heraclides of Tarentum (*fl.* third to second century BC), Archigenes (*fl.* first to second century AD) and Criton (second century AD), physician to the wife of Trajan, Plotina. In his discussion of such authors, Galen (12.445–446 Kühn 1826) makes it clear that he deems writings on cosmetics to be an embarrassment, particularly for doctors.

The Hippocratic text, *Diseases of Women* (1.106), has two recipes for removal of body hair: (i) grapevine sap and oil, and (ii) burnt and pounded *alcyonea* (cf. pp. 71–74) diluted with wine. In the same section the author also recommends applying oil to the eye area after plucking, indicating that women shaped their eyebrows. There is also a remedy for hair loss that includes pigeon dung and nettles (2.189). This recipe, situated amid medical treatments, again exemplifies the idea that cosmeceuticals for conditions affecting one's appearance were legitimate concerns of doctors. Theophrastus's *On Odours* discusses perfumes in detail – also uncontroversially and within a scientific framework of enquiry – and *Enquiry into Plants* 9.7 is devoted to the same. The direct association between perfumes and feminine beautification did not concern Theophrastus, whose works reflect the medical tradition that aligned sweet smells with good health (to promote it and as a symptom of it). This tradition was continued by later writers such as Dioscorides (first century AD) who were educated in the medical benefits of perfumes, particularly in the healing of sores and open wounds.

There are also extensive archaeological records that attest to the widespread use of cosmetics and cosmeceuticals. Cleanliness was important, particularly among the Roman elite, and the maintenance of personal hygiene included bathing and the use of oil-based soaps and exfoliants. Extensive remains of public baths such as the Stabian Baths at Pompeii reveal a highly ordered bathing routine. Although the women's area is smaller than the men's baths, the architecture shows several separate spaces, including waiting rooms and changing rooms. Balsdon (1962: 267) suggests that the baths also included beauty parlours and treatment rooms,[6] as attested by Seneca the Younger's reference to the noises coming from a bath near his house, which included the cries of men being plucked (*Epistle* 56).

Wealthier Romans could bathe at home where they were afforded privacy and also protection from the side-effects of washing in other people's water. Bathing was not only for maintaining hygiene, and thereby recommended by various physicians,[7] it was also associated with beautification. Feminine adornment scenes attest to the pivotal role of bathing from as early as the Homeric age (cf. *Iliad* 14.166ff.) and are regularly depicted in both Greek and Roman artwork with a focus on Aphrodite / Venus at her bath in heady representations of hygiene, beautification and eroticism.

After bathing, some Romans applied a deodorant (cf. p. 116) and cleaned their teeth (cf. pp. 117–119). They may have also applied certain unguents or lotions to soothe the skin, relieving any irritation and restoring moisture. Such substances, like cosmetics, were kept in various containers, usually called *pyxides*, made of bronze, ceramic, glass, silver and even ivory, mostly cylindrical in shape with a separate lid. Plain *pyxides* are common archaeological finds (Fig. 1), as are more ornate ones that may have also served as display pieces on dressing tables (Fig. 2). The contents of such containers were extracted with specialized tools, many indistinguishable from medical implements, which took the form of spatulas, tiny spoons and phials. These objects, along with combs (Figs 3, 5 and 6), hair pins and other forms of adornment such as jewellery were categorized by Livy (34.7) and Varro (*De Lingua Latina* 5.29.129) as the *mundus muliebris* ('woman's toilette'). An excellent example of the *mundus muliebris* is the well-preserved cosmetic box from Campania that houses all sorts of beauty accoutrements, including a bronze mirror (cf. Fig. 3 and also p. 122).

Mirrors provided a means of monitoring the beautification process, ensuring that all the steps of enhancement were followed for a successful result. Ovid is aware of the significance of the mirror in the *mundus muliebris*. He instructs women to consult their mirrors before they embark on a particular hairstyle (*AA* 3.135–136); predicts the sorrow that will inevitably come to every woman when she looks at her mirror (*Med. ll.*45–48); suggests to a newly bald Corinna to avoid gazing at herself (*Am.* 1.14.37–38); and even advises the would-be lover to hold his mistress's mirror for her (*AA* 2.215–216). The erotic connotations of feminine adornment are attested by the decorative scenes depicted upon mirrors; for example, the three Graces (Fig. 4),[8] Venus, scenes of sexual congress, and myths such as Leda and the swan and Europa and the bull (further on the mirror, cf. Bartsch 2006; Wyke 1994).

Yet mirrors were also depicted in funerary reliefs of respectable women, namely those *matronae* ('matrons') who had embodied the esteemed value of *pudicitia* while they were alive. Such reliefs, often accompanied by other adornment motifs, may have been intended to signify familial wealth, but perhaps also to testify to individual women's refinement and circumspect sense of style.[9] Taylor (2008: 35) suggests that there is no anomaly in such monuments: 'Bourgeois respectability, it seems, went in for common taste; many were the Roman women who preferred to be immortalized with some material reminiscence of their daily toilette. Even the mirror could be presented as an adjunct to matronly chastity.'

There is also a surfeit of archaeological evidence for hair adornment. Numerous hair ornaments and more functional pieces such as pins have been found in public baths – trapped in drains and secreted in other places – along

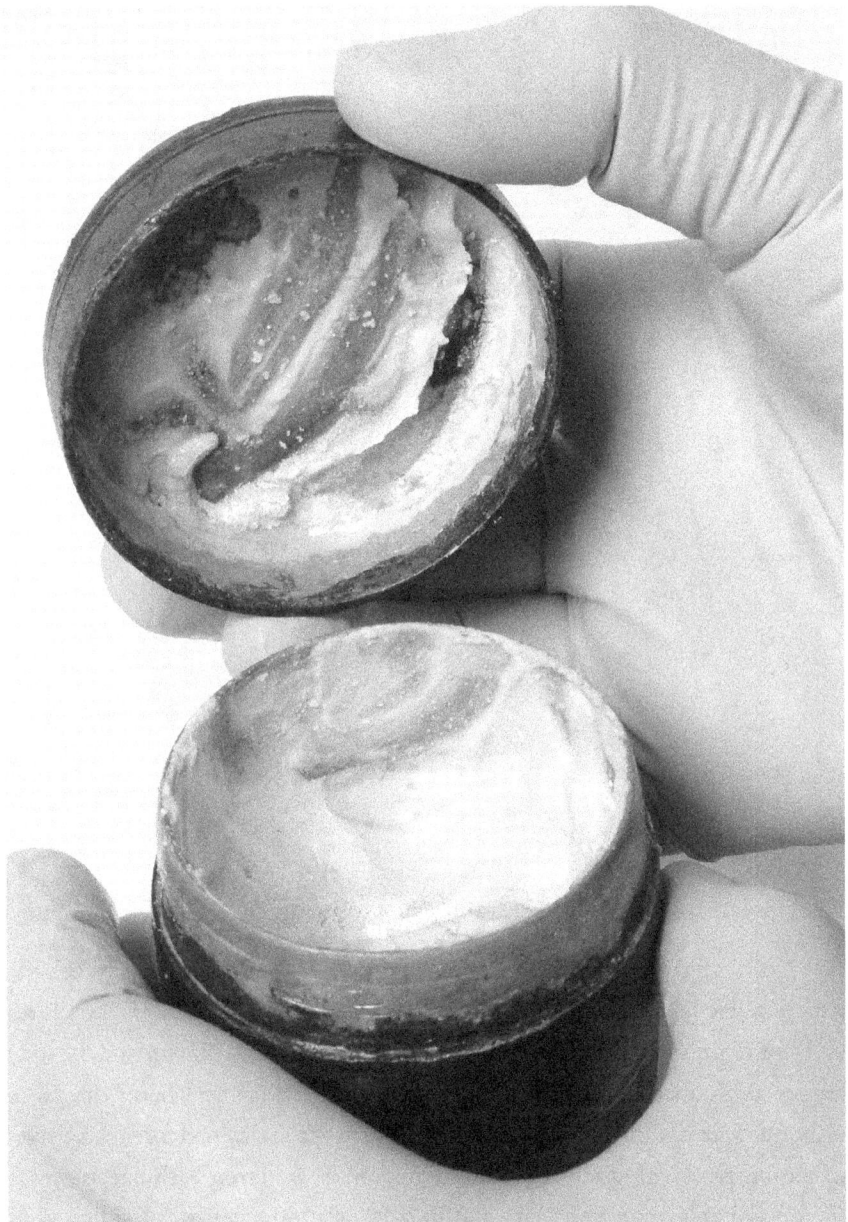

**Fig. 1** Roman container with cosmeceutical cream. Mid-second century AD.

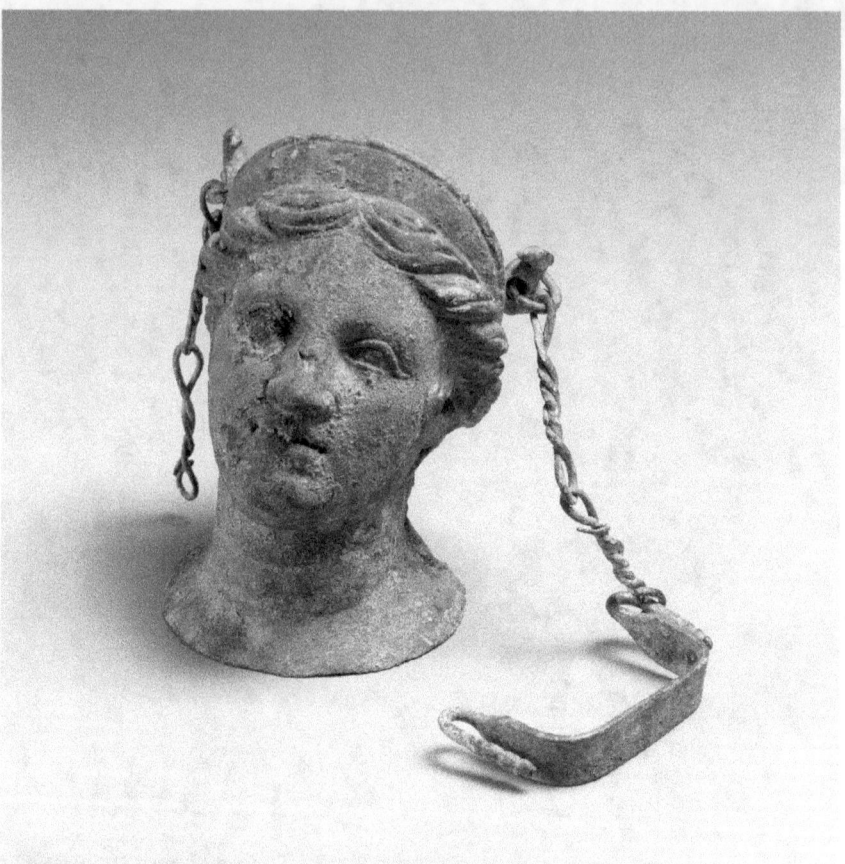

**Fig. 2** Bronze cosmetics container. Fourth to third century BC.

with jewellery and other items. Official portraits, decorative frescoes, sculptures and coins provide evidence for various hairdos, which Bartman (2001: 1) argues 'reproduce real styles that could be made with real hair.' The more elaborate styles of the Flavian era and later, such as the elevated forehead crown of pin-curls adorning the Fonseca Bust, could be achieved with hair pieces if there were a dearth of one's natural hair. Wigs and hairpieces, mentioned in written sources, have not fared as well as other material artefacts, except in Egypt where discoveries show a markedly different hair aesthetic compared to Roman styles. Additionally, while we know both women and men used dye, unlike the occasional deposits left in cosmetic jars, no equivalent traces of hair colourants are extant.

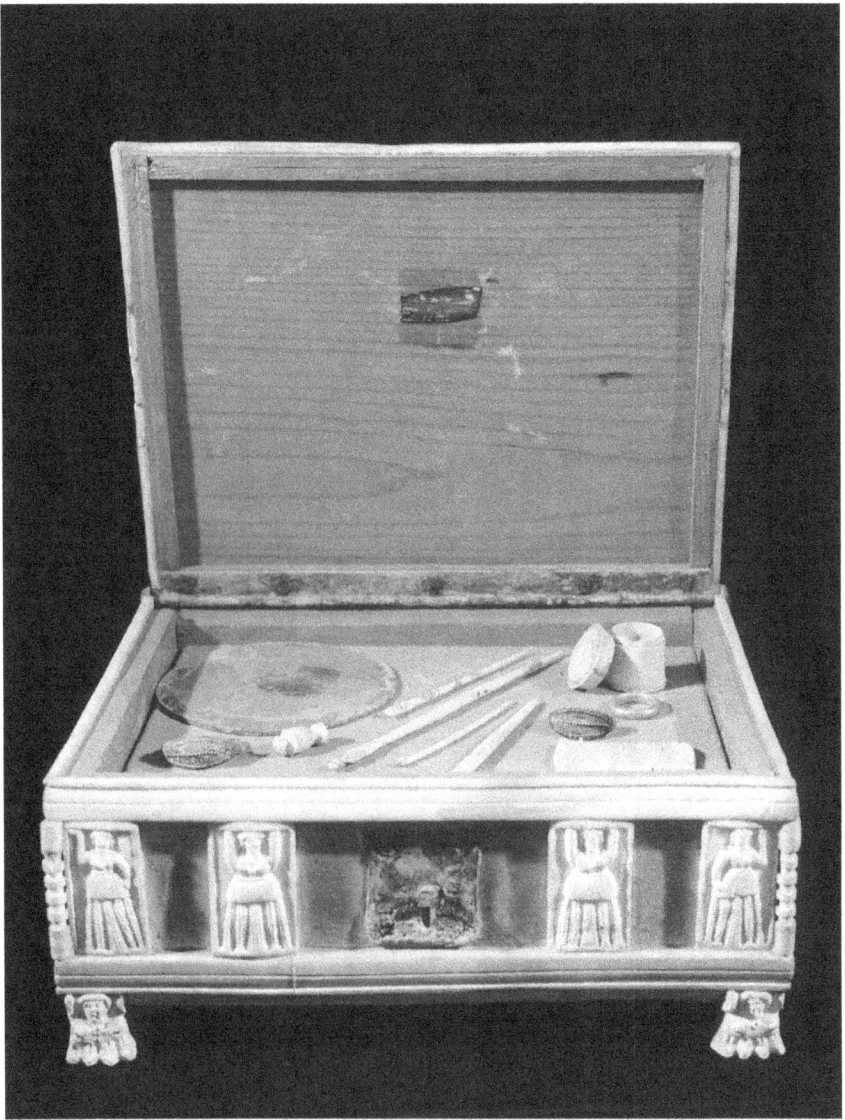

Fig. 3 Box containing toiletries, from Cumae, Campania. First century AD.

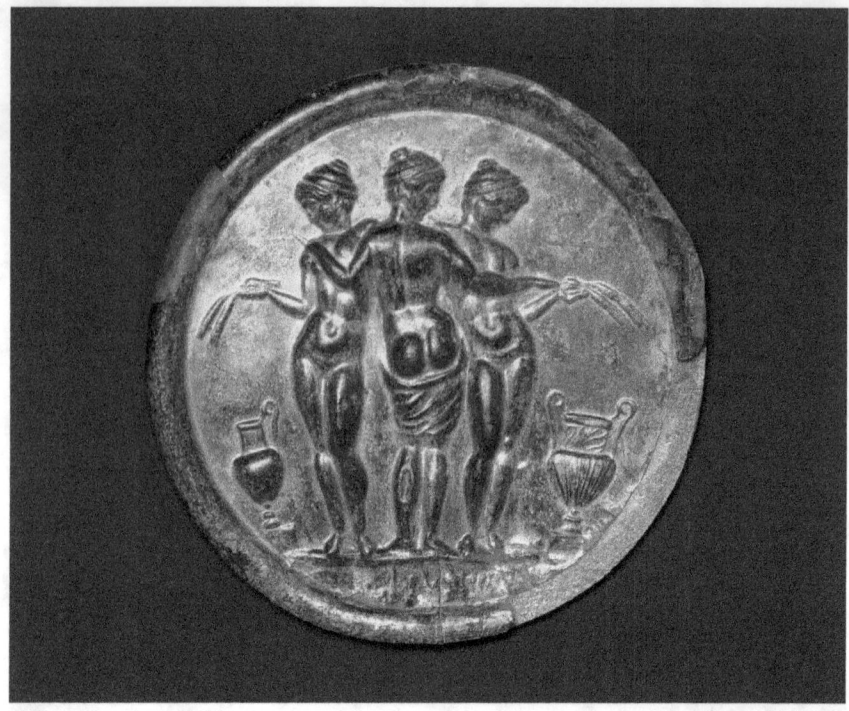

**Fig. 4** Gilded bronze mirror depicting the Three Graces. Second century AD.

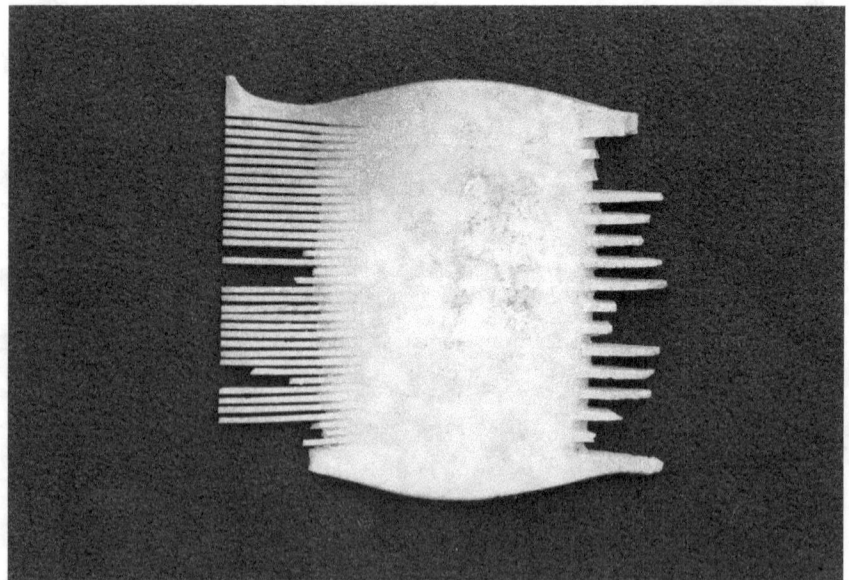

**Fig. 5** Roman double-sided ivory comb. First century BC to second century AD.

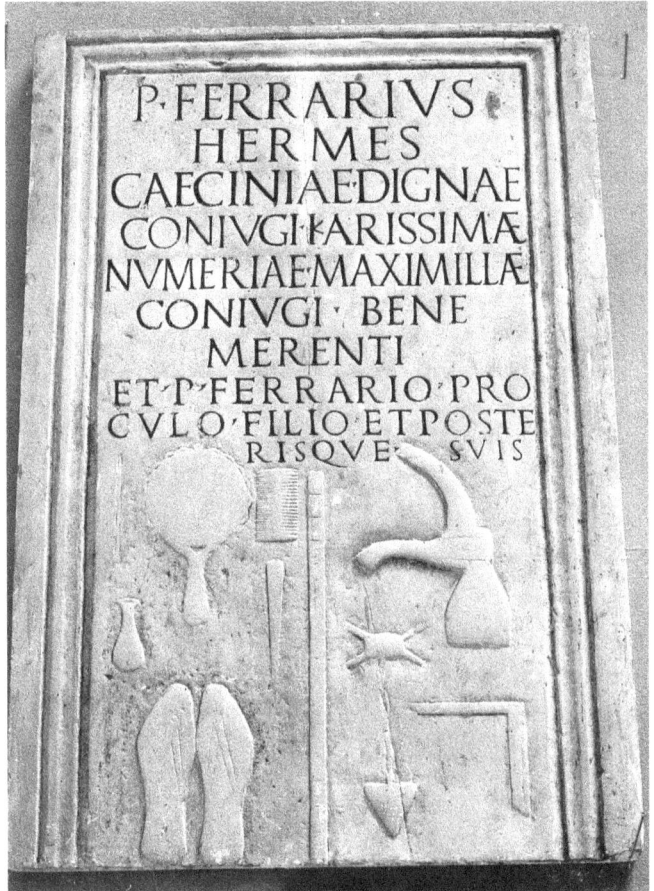

**Fig. 6** Stele of P. Ferrarius Hermes. First century BC to second century AD.

## Ovid on *cultus*, *munditia* and *ars*

Three of the four texts under analysis herein belong to the middle period of Ovid's literary career. As Toohey (2013: 157) remarks: 'Ovid's didactic poems were published in quick succession' and all three of the erotodidactic works – the *Medicamina*, *Ars Amatoria* and *Remedia* – follow on closely from the second edition of the *Amores*. In this respect, the *Amores*, published as late as 3 BC in its revised form, may be regarded as being on the cusp of the middle period, thereby providing a smooth segue to the erotodidactic collection. Indeed, Ovid references the *Amores* in the didactic works through the unconventional choice of the elegiac couplet, which defines them as both instructional and erotic. A characteristic of Ovid's erotodidactic works is the tripartite system of *cultus-munditia-ars* and it is through this paradigm that he is able to explore feminine beautification (usually) free from opprobrium and express his philosophies on cultivation and simple elegance.

*cultus* is 'labour' or 'care' and in the process of *cultus*, one renders something improved, refined or, in effect, cultivated. It is therefore aligned with progress and civilization in relation to land, shelter, society and the individual. In relation to society, *cultus* marks a developed urban environment in contrast to one that is rustic and lacking in the sophisticated markers of cultural evolution. In an advanced society, the sophisticates participate in the process of self-improvement, applying the precepts of *cultus* to educate the mind, perfect etiquette and enhance appearance. *cultus* thereby competes with nature because it alters it in order to improve upon it.

In the Ovidian schema of adornment, *cultus* is linked with *munditia* and *ars*. As discussed above, the Romans associated beauty and beauty treatments with hygiene. Cleanliness was encapsulated in the term *munditia*, which also designates neatness, style, and simple elegance.[10] The malleability and inclusiveness evoked by this word, as with *cultus*, ensured that its use to describe a woman's self-presentation denoted an overall package: clean skin, hair and breath; a fresh smell; stylish clothing, make-up and accessories. Gibson (2006: 126), who regards Ovid's views on such matters as decidedly moderate, particularly in the *Ars*, observes the distinction between the poet's position and that of the moralists, writing on *AA* 3.129–134:

> The wearing of costly jewellery and expensive clothing is regularly regarded by moralists in opposition to personal simplicity. Ovid's female pupils are likewise warned to eschew *luxuria*. But it is clear from Ovid's earlier and provocative 'hymn' to *cultus* (101–34), and from instruction which follows in *Ars* 3 on hairstyles, clothing, and cosmetics, that Ovid does not accept that his pupils must therefore travel to the opposite 'extreme' of simplicity. In any case, the ground of Ovid's opposition to jewellery and clothing differs from that of the moralists. The latter saw in these items evidence of corrupting *luxuria*, while for Ovid they lack the qualities of taste and elegance (*munditiae*). That is to say, what for others is a matter of ethics, for Ovid is aesthetics: such displays of wealth repel lovers.

The moderation that characterizes Ovid's use of *munditia* also underlies his concept of *cultus*. Ovid does not extol the luxury associated with *cultus*, except when it clearly suits a particular rhetorical imperative (cf. pp. 52–53), and in this sense, he offers a unique understanding of the women of Augustan Rome. Rather than the simplicities of the idealized *matronae* of epic and historical texts, or the *meretrices* and the *puellae* ('girls', 'girlfriends') of the elegiac poets, or even the ghastly hybrids of the wife-whore of satire, Ovid's women are sophisticated, classy, well-groomed urbanites.

The key to achieving this style, a combination of Ovidian *cultus* and *munditia*, is the application of Ovidian *ars*. Therefore, in the *Medicamina*, beauty can be improved upon and maintained by the application of carefully prepared cosmeceuticals. While some of the ingredients in the lotions are expensive and thus luxurious, Ovid also lists less costly items. The cheaper alternatives to expensive fabrics in *Ars* Book Three, for example, suggest that with an eye for a bargain and a skilled sense of style, non-elite women could also afford the markers of *cultus*.[11]

Another important aspect of *ars* is privacy and secrecy. The processes of beautification are not to be shared, particularly with one's partner, for the revelation of such is inimical to the very 'point' of beautification. While this is not discussed in the extant lines of the *Medicamina*, it is explained in both *AA* 3.209–234 and *Rem.* ll.343–356. In Ovid's system of beautification, *ars* is a trick or a deceit, which by alignment with *cultus* and *munditia*, is necessary for female refinement and sophistication. The women of Ovid's era, unlike the unsubtle courtesans of Alexis's *Isostasion*, who may look presentable from a distance, are more like the masterpieces of Myron (*AA* 3.219) or intricate jewellery that glitters and impresses (*AA* 3.221, 223–224). And, like such markers of civilization, they must only be unveiled when they are complete.

While Ovid usually presents an open, relaxed and somewhat egalitarian attitude to female adornment, he is not always as cavalier when it comes to issues of male *cultus*. As *AA* 1.505–524 illustrates, Ovid's opinions on male beautification can be traditional and reactionary. For a Roman male, a natural body was a culturally familiar and culturally approved body and one aligned with accepted and expected moralities. For a man to transcend the physical boundaries that segregated his body from the female via adoption of gender markers culturally assigned to women was to flirt with *mollitia* ('softness', 'effeminacy' and 'voluptuousness') and the social stigma attached to it. As Edwards (2002: 68) explains: 'The victim of the accusation [of *mollitia*] is alleged to be over-careful in his dress, often affecting "feminine" and/or exotic clothes.... The "effeminate" man is perfumed, bathes more often than is necessary and depilates his legs.' *mollitia* is, therefore, not to be encouraged, even by Ovid, who, in the aforementioned passage from *Ars* Book One, dissuades men from curling their hair and smoothing their legs. His recommendation for masculine appeal privileges *munditia*; a 'look' akin to carefully styled ruggedness.

At *Med.* ll.23–26, however, there is a different attitude expressed, with an emphasis on *cultus* in a vivid evocation of the dapper men of the Augustan age. Partly a picture of well-groomed men (*ll.*23–24) and partly a comic jibe at their expense (*ll.*25–26), these lines show the Ovid of the *Medicamina* as a man of moderation with a keen sense of taste. Here Ovid's persona is that of the urbane sophisticate; a man who possesses a liberal attitude to male beautification with a touch of wry amusement.

Turning to *cultus* and related themes in the *Amores* we find Ovid to be relatively quiet. Nevertheless, the few references show the early stages of his philosophy on adornment. In *Am.* 2.10.5 he claims that the two women he loves are both *formosa* ('beautiful') and endowed with *cultus*. Similarly, in *Am.* 3.7.1, he uses *formosa* and *cultus* to describe a desirable woman. In *Am.* 3.4.37–42 there is also an attempt at defining *cultus* through an indirect contrast with *rusticus* ('rustic') when Ovid uses the latter of an overly protective husband[12] who is offended at his *adultera coniunx* ('adulterous wife'). While *cultus* is not named, as a strong antonym of *rusticus*, it is implicit (cf. *AA* 3.127–128 for the juxtaposition of the two terms).

## Ovid and Augustus's moral legislation

The brief consideration of *cultus* in the *Amores* (above) shows occasions of Ovid's amoral attitude towards sexuality and, in the case of *Am.* 3.4, his defiance of the *lex Iulia de adulteriis coercendis*. The law, introduced by Augustus in 18 BC, aimed to promote marriage and the birth of legitimate children, and consequently forbade sexual activities such as adultery, principally illicit relations with married women, be they divorcees or even widows. Other poems in the collection that overtly address adultery are 2.19 (a companion poem to 3.4), 3.8 and 3.12. Ovid presents himself in the *Amores* as a decadent who appears to pursue erotic encounters free from any restraints, including that of class or social standing. He enjoys Corinna (*Am.* 1.5); he has sex with her hairdresser, Cypassis (*Am.* 2.8); he chides men who seek to protect their women, of whatever status; he is a slave to Cupid's power (*Am.* 1.1, 1.2, 3.9); he sees *amor* as a battle (*Am.* 1.9, 2.9); and even admits defeat (*Am.* 3.7). Not surprisingly, the cavalier attitude of the *Amores*, and the inherent indifference to the reforms of Augustus, have prompted scholars such as Davis (1999: 449) to regard the collection as equally controversial as the *Ars Amatoria*:

> Whereas in the *Ars Amatoria* the poet at least gestures towards defending himself against the charge of promoting adultery, in the *Amores* he openly presents himself as an adulterer. Augustus exiled Ovid to Tomis because of the *Ars Amatoria*. He might equally have banished him for writing the *Amores*.

One may in fact conjecture that the collection is more controversial except that it lacks one integral ingredient: unlike the *Ars*, it is not a handbook promoting un-Roman activities.

In the first two collections of the erotodidactic period, Ovid's celebrations of *cultus* are particularly antithetical to another Augustan precept, namely the promotion of traditional attire and modesty in self-presentation. Ovid's position on adornment and consumption in the *Medicamina* and the *Ars* is, therefore, additionally provocative. This is exacerbated in the *Medicamina* because all women are free to enjoy the poem, and thus, by default, encouraged to delight in the material benefits of a healthy Italian economy and a robust trade market.[13] There remains only one caveat: remember that inner integrity and good taste are integral parts of *cultus*. As Rosati (1985: 30–32) and Gibson (2003: 145) have commented, the emphasis on esteemed behaviour and inner fortitude, implicitly linked with *cultus* in the *Medicamina*, demonstrates Ovid's championing of feminine cultivation as something that can be practised without rejecting traditional societal values and respectability.

Despite an uncensored audience and a comparatively liberal attitude to female adornment, both of which Augustus may well have found irritating (despite the caveat), the *Medicamina* is mild in comparison to the *Ars Amatoria*, which strays regularly into matters sexual and, by default, illegal. Ovid begins the *Ars* nobly enough, taking care to issue warnings that the collection is restricted; in *AA* 1.31–34, for example, he plays with Augustus's encouragement of the wearing of the *stola* ('robe') and *vittae* ('headbands') for *matronae*:

> este procul, vittae tenues, insigne pudoris,
>   quaeque tegis medios instita longa pedes:
> nos Venerem tutam concessaque furta canemus
>   inque meo nullum carmine crimen erit.

> Away, slim headbands [*vittae*], signs of modesty [*pudor*],
>   and you long tunic trailing down past the ankles:
> I sing of safe Venus and permissible amours
>   and in my song will be no crime.

These lines clarify Ovid's intended audience in Book One and, consequently, the other two Books (cf. 2.599–600; 3.57–58, 483, 613–616), by alluding to those women who are *not* his intended audience: *matronae*.[14] Dress is important here; Ovid designates his intended readers as *meretrices* – women socially identified by their clothing – namely, the *toga*, not the *stola* and *palla*.[15] In *Ars* Book Three, a female-oriented text, Ovid again makes it clear that *matronae* are not the intended audience, specifying that he is composing for 'she' who has been recently liberated from the rod (*l*.361). Earlier, at *ll*.57–58, he states that in respect to the audience of the Book, he is alert to the *lex Iulia* and to those women who, under its strictures, are permitted a degree of licence (that it, *meretrices*). The audience is, therefore, ostensibly comprised of *libertinae* ('freedwomen'), which clearly included *meretrices*. *libertinae*, however, is a slippery term. Griffin (1976: 103) encapsulates the ambiguities: 'Between *libertinae* and ἑταῖραι [*hetairai*], between actresses and *meretrices*, even between some professionals and some *matronae*, the dividing line cannot have been so easy to draw as in theory, perhaps, it should have been.' Additionally, Volk (2006: 238) points out:

> This picture is somewhat complicated by the fact that there is no evidence that freedwomen were exempted from the strictures of the *lex Iulia* – which

does raise the question of what women Ovid really thinks he is teaching and whether he can possibly be sincere in his avowed adherence to the Augustan laws.

There are clearly problems, then, with Ovid's disclaimers, despite his later attempts in Book Three to 'interpret' the law as exempting all freedwomen (cf. *ll*.611–658).[16] But the glitches and complications extend much further than fluidity of categories and legal ambiguities.[17] Watson (2002: 156) makes some pragmatically insightful observations that further contradict Ovid's stated claims not to be composing for a chaste, socially elite female audience, beginning with the obvious point that didactic teaching is not necessarily 'directed solely at the addressee of the poem', and further:

> There are many indications that Ovid had *matronae* in mind. For instance, allusions to activities such as wool-making (2.686) and frequent childbirth (3.81–82) are more appropriate to married women than to courtesans. The use of the famous Mars/Venus love affair – an unequivocal case of adultery – as an exemplum has been commented on.

As for the *Remedia*, Ovid's focus on, or interaction with, the Augustan regime is characterized by a defensive stance in relation to the negative reception of the *Ars Amatoria*. The defence takes the form of a digression at *Rem*. 361–396 in which Ovid references detractors who have called the collection *proterva* ('shameless', *l*.362). The digression may well include a not-so-veiled swipe at Augustus, or at least a fulsome resentment of him and his rules, as indicated by *ll*.389–392, particularly the exclamatory words of *l*.389: *rumpere, Livor edax* ('burst, greedy Spite'). In the illuminating article by Casali (2006), the *Remedia* is interpreted as Ovid's swan song to poetic games involving the *lex Iulia* and the moral platform of the *principate* in general. What these witticisms, mixed messages and, at times, outright subversions are replaced with are one more didactic elegy, the *Fasti*, Ovid's calendar cast as military service to Augustus (2.9), roughly coinciding with the *Metamorphoses*, followed by the poems of despair and repentance. It is no coincidence, then, that the *Remedia* farewells the fun of the erotodidactic collection in the nastiest of ways, as the *praeceptor* becomes the doctor, metaphorically returning to his model Nicander (cf. p. 25), whose works set out to heal the deadliest of bites. As Nicander instructs on removing snake venom, Ovid instructs on healing the wounds of *amor* (cf. Watson 2002: 163). Rightly, the poets seeks the assistance of Apollo and his gift of healing (*Rem.* 75–78).

## The texts

The following discussion provides introductory detail with attention to the sources of Ovid's inspiration. As his allusions, imitations and homages are assembled from a vast literary repertoire, the focus is a particularly selective one: didactic genres for the *Medicamina*; the poet's immediate elegiac predecessors, Tibullus and Propertius, for the *Amores*, plus Callimachus and Catullus for Alexandrian and neoteric inspiration respectively; a return to didactic works in the form of 'pillow-books' and illustrated sex manuals for the *Ars Amatoria*; and satire for the *Remedia*. All of these neatly packaged genres, poets and authors filter throughout almost every one of Ovid's poems to greater and lesser extents and bring with them numerous colleagues and compositions. The examples offered below are, therefore, a drop in the literary ocean.

### *Medicamina Faciei Femineae*

The *Medicamina* (c. 2 BC)[18] is a unique work in Roman literature, not only because it offers a counterbalance to the anti-cosmetic tradition and presents a more nuanced view of feminine cultivation, but because it is aimed at women and of specific interest to them. Most of the few publications on the work focus on its didactic nature, yet its sensual qualities are also important. Dispensing with the hexametric tradition of instructional poetry and adopting the elegiac metre of the *Amores*, Ovid speaks to his female audience on an intimate topic in an intimate manner.[19] Thus he adopts the authorial pose of the teacher of women that echoes the persona of the *lena* ('procuress') whose role, among other things, is to prettify women for sex with clients (cf. Myers 1996; Watson 2001).

Ovid's awareness of the erotic nature of the metre, and his promotion of this, are conveyed in his personification of Elegy as emphatically feminine and sensual in *Am.* 3.1.7–10:

Venit odoratos Elegia nexa capillos,
   et, puto, pes illi longior alter erat.
Forma decens, vestis tenuissima, vultus amantis,
   et pedibus vitium causa decoris erat.

Elegy comes with scented locks bound,
   and, I believe, one foot was longer than the other.
Her appearance was becoming, her dress most delicate, her expression affectionate,
   and the imperfection with her feet was the source of her charm.

Assisted by this sensual metre, Ovid metaphorically enters the female chamber in the *Medicamina*, as he writes of woman's flesh and poetically touches woman's face and body. Like the poetic embodiment of Amor, sometimes depicted alongside the female at her toilette in Roman art,[20] Ovid cultivates female skin, instructs and assists in beautification and holds an elegiac mirror for woman to gaze at the finished product. The demarcation point of privacy and secrecy that traditionally marginalizes the woman at her toilette is thereby breached by Ovid in a poetic exercise that traverses gendered segregation.[21]

Ovid's intimacy is also tempered with down-to-earth instruction befitting didactic poetry. The technicality of traditional didactic poetry begins at *l.*51, which is a salient reminder to modern readers that *ll.*1–50 constitute a proem to what was originally a longer work. While the exact length of the original poem remains uncertain, the substantial introductory passage has been interpreted by Toohey (2013: 162) as indicative of a length of some 800 lines. In contrast, Watson (2002: 142), noting Ovid's description of the *Medicamina* as *parvus* ('small') at *AA*. 3.205, suggests something closer to Virgil's *Georgics* ('a piece that Ovid certainly had in mind'), which places the length at around 500 lines. Ovid's use of the term *parvus*, however, may be nothing more than a pseudo-bashful conceit, similar in tone to Catullus's description of his poems as *nugae* ('trifles') at 1.4. The possibility of an ironic tone, however, is not mutually exclusive to Watson's suggested length, particularly in view of the subject matter, which may have proven tiresome if excessively long.

Despite the usual regret expressed by scholars at the loss of ancient texts, Ovid's broken *Medicamina* has not always been met with lament.[22] The robust dismissal by Wilkinson (1995: 118) is particularly memorable:

The subject chosen by Ovid was cosmetics (*medicamina faciei*), and after fifty clever and spirited lines of introductions he plunges into a series of versified recipes, presumably taken from some prose treatise by a professional pharmacologist. It is hardly a matter of regret that after a further fifty lines our manuscripts break off. One would like to think that Ovid broke off too. He tells us that the book was small, but he also indicates that it was published ... What can have induced him to embark on such a poem? He was not a tasteless bore, as Nicander (to judge from his two extant verse treatises) most certainly was.

In addition to characterizations of the work as either boring or trivial or both, there has been limited scholarly attention paid to the *Medicamina*. The publication of Rosati's edition with extensive notes in 1985 has gone some way to legitimizing research on the work, and Watson (2001) and Rimell (2005 and 2006) have followed with insightful analyses. Prior to these studies, Green (1979) provided a detailed discussion of the recipes and addressed the significance of the work in extending approaches to Ovid's views on women, the didactic genre and the persona of the *praeceptor amoris*.[23] As these studies have shown, the *Medicamina* may be a parodic and incongruous example of didactic literature (cf. Toohey 2013: 161; Watson 2001; Watson 2002: 146–147), but it is far from mediocre. It may not have the spectacle of the *Metamorphoses*, or the intensity and haunting beauty of the *Tristia*, or even the delightful variations and erotic daring of the *Ars*, but in the context of its genre and subject matter, it is informative and interesting.

While the subject matter may be regarded as frivolous, it is not without precedent, and Ovid shows himself to be a poet who pays deference to his artistic heritage. Watson (2001: 458) has discussed the links to 'the subgenre of didactic poems (*artes*) on non-serious subjects, such as those composed for the Saturnalia'. In the *Tristia* 2.471–490, as Watson notes, Ovid provides a defence of poetry on such trivial subjects, describing works on dice and various board games, swimming instruction and painting (2.487). Such works, Ovid argues, are the subjects of play in the month of December (2.491), which references the Saturnalia and the provision of 'gift' books for amusement. At 2.493 Ovid acknowledges that such spirited didactic literature furnished the inspiration behind some of his own collections – works that were neither stern nor gloomy – but that, nevertheless, resulted in punishment.

Ovid was also influenced by more serious didactic poetry as well as technical prose works on medicine, cosmeceuticals and cosmetics from the Alexandrian age. The enthusiasm for didactic poetry during this period resulted in several innovations, including the liberation of subject matter to incorporate the trivial and comic, an emphasis on the ludic capabilities of didacticism and explorations of, and experiments in, the transformative effects of metaphrastic exercises (cf. Callimachus's adoption of the elegiac metre for his *Aetia*).[24] Extant examples of metaphrastic didactic include the *Phaenomena* of Aratus (*c.* 315–240 BC), a poem on star-signs and weather-signs, based on a prose text by Eudoxus and possibly a work by Theophrastus, and the *Theriaca* and *Alexipharmaca* of Nicander (*fl.* second century BC). Despite Wilkinson's dismissal of Nicander as a bore, his work influenced Ovid in various ways and in view of the subject matter of the *Theriaca* and *Alexipharmaca* – venomous creatures and remedies for their bites, and poisons and antidotes, respectively – they are lively and fascinating reads. What makes them so, and what would have appealed to Ovid, are Nicander's occasional liking for the gruesome, his random outbursts of sensationalism (described by Toohey (2013: 62) as similar to a style 'normally reserved for tabloid newspapers'), and the ludic qualities of his writing that are frequently expressed in obscurities of vocabulary and metaphor. Indeed, Nicander's wild flourishes, exhilarating descriptions of the effects of poisons, mythological *exempla* and heroic similes, interspersed with instruction, mark his works as precursors to both the *Medicamina* and also the *Metamorphoses*.[25]

Of the Roman writers, Ovid's primary source of imitation is Virgil's *Georgics*. The allusions are, as Watson (2001: 461) states, designed to raise the theme of the *Medicamina* to the important level of agriculture, 'legitimising it as a subject for a didactic poem'. The immediate point of poetic debt is evidenced in Ovid's treatment of *cultus* and its relationship to *cura*, which is reminiscent of certain Virgilian passages, such as 2.35–37:

Quare agite o proprios generatim discite cultus,
agricolae, fructusque feros mollite colendo,
neu segnes iaceant terrae.

Wherefore come, farmers, learn the cultivation [*cultus*] appropriate to

> each species, by cultivation [*colere*] tame the wild fruits,
> that the earth should not lie idle.

As Virgil writes of cultivation to soften wild fruit and prevent fallow land, Ovid eulogizes *cultus* for similar reasons. Virgil extends his definition of *cultus* to embrace human achievements in the realms of engineering and architecture in his famous eulogy to Italy in *Georgics* 2.136–176, which recalls the praise of Italy's fertile soil in Varro's *De Res Rustica* 1.2.3–7. Again, this is matched by Ovid's segue from agriculture to civilization at *Med. ll.*7–10, which includes *cultus* in the form of golden halls and marble monuments. The *Georgics*, like the *Medicamina*, also acknowledges the benefits of an expansive empire in relation to the importation of the markers of *cultus*. In *Georgics* 1.56–57, Virgil lists saffron fragrance from Lydia, ivory from India and incense from Arabia; foreshadowing Ovid's references to imported luxuries such as Indian ivory (*Med. l.*10) and gems from the East (*Med. l.*21).

Virgil also includes plant knowledge that reveals his use of Theophrastus's *Enquiry into Plants*. In Book Four, Theophrastus focuses on the influence of environment and climate on plant and tree species, which Virgil references in *Georgics* 2.109–135. A more direct textual parallel occurs at *Georgics* 2.56–59 on the benefits derived from the Median citron[26] where Virgil cites two of the same benefits of the plant as listed by Theophrastus at 4.2 (its use as an antidote to poison as well as a mouth-freshener). The imitation of Theophrastus's didactic prose shows a shared poetic practice between Virgil and Ovid in their adoption of poetic renderings of Alexandrian technical treatises.[27]

There are also significant points of poetic departure between the *Georgics* and the *Medicamina*, which reflect the different political and social climates in which they were composed, as well as different artistic imperatives. Otis (1970: 1–2) has stressed the need to recognize Ovid as an artist from 'a wholly different Augustan generation'; an approach revived by Habinek (2002: 46) as an important interpretive consideration when assessing not only these two poets, but the Augustan poets per se (cf. also Tarrant 2013: 14). Whereas Virgil's work, in part, reflects the newly (re)founded Rome with its ties to, and dependence upon, a past characterized by *labor* and *industria*; Ovid's work reflects the developed *principate* as an institution of revision that addressed and reshaped constructions of political authority, religion and cult, as well as sexuality and gender. Virgil was witness to the rise of Augustan Rome but Ovid lived in it.

This generational difference is perhaps why there are moments of uncertainty in the *Georgics* in relation to *cultus* that are absent from the *Medicamina*. In Book Two in 'The Praise of the Farmer' (*ll*.458–542), Virgil returns to images of unprompted or uncultivated earthly bounties and juxtaposes them to images of cultivated luxury in the form of mansions, lavish clothing and other exotica. Here Virgil promotes the quietude and peace of a life free of deceit (*natura* transformed into *cultus* transformed into *luxuria*). In contrast, the *Medicamina* shows no such anxieties as Ovid records the women of his age making the most of the bounties of empire; as Habinek (2002: 50) states:

> Here the age-old anxieties about women as consumers ... are cast aside in favour of a celebration of the imperial cornucopia. Sumptuary laws and other strategies of élite 'auto-conservation' are unnecessary in the new global economy. *Cultus* becomes an end in itself, whether it's planting, pruning, grafting, covering, or dyeing – your face.

The tensions between Virgil and Ovid's responses to *cultus* and the generation 'gap' between them in regard to the evolution of the *principate*, succinctly expressed by Habinek in his summation of Ovid's agenda, are also present in the prooemium of the *Medicamina*. As discussed above, Ovid echoes the *Georgics* here, and Watson (2001: 467) argues for a 'mock-serious' tone and an attitude that is 'subversive (at least playfully, if not maliciously) of the ideology espoused in the *Georgics* and of Augustan ideology in general.'

## *Amores*

Originally composed over a decade before the *Medicamina*, with its latest publication date merely a year or so before it, the *Amores* is a celebrated rejection of epic in favour of the amorous, playful and emotional genre of elegy. The decision to write elegy is a motif of the collection and is presaged as such in the opening poem of Book One. Ovid explains that he started with epic but was disturbed by Cupid who compelled him to write elegy instead. In other poems in the collection he further explains that elegy also came in the form of the inspirational women around him, including Corinna (*Am.* 2.1, 2.12 and 2.18) who, coincidentally embodies key facets of the evocative image of the goddess Elegy of *Am.* 3.1.7–20 (on the motif, cf. also *Am.* 3.1, 3.8 and 3.9).

In comparison to the *Medicamina* and as traditional elegy rather than didactic or erotodidactic poetry, the *Amores* presents the reader with a different authorial pose – indeed there are several 'authors' speaking in the collection – and a different audience. The primary role adopted by Ovid is, obviously, that of the *amator* ('lover'), but his is a most versatile, chameleon-like *amator* who shares a variety of experiences – celebratory, embarrassing and painful – and voices a variety of opinions on *amor* that are not necessarily consistent. The likelihood of an intended female audience, with the possible exception of *meretrices*, seems out of the question, and the memorable description of Ovid's readership proffered by Greene (1994: 349) still remains one of the best: '[an] audience of sexually excitable (perhaps predatory) men.' Ovid therefore writes for 'himself' in 'others', that is, with an understanding that his readers will be thoughtful in their responses to his themes, able to appreciate them and to see themselves mirrored therein. Thus the *Amores* not only foreshadows the metre and amatory concerns of the *Medicamina* and the *Ars*, it also predates and anticipates the jilted lovers for whom the *Remedia* is composed.

In *Am.* 1.15.9–30, Ovid provides a list of immortal authors and while he does not claim them as direct influences, their names evoke his literary learning and sources of homage and imitation. From this list, the most immediate and named influence is Tibullus. While Propertius is curiously absent, he is the primary influence on *Amores* overall and this very poem in particular (emphasized by Ovid's imitation of Propertius 2.34.27–45 in this sweeping evocation of authors). In this instance acknowledgement is best suited to imitation rather than naming.

Both Propertius and Tibullus influenced Ovid's *Amores* in their joint establishment of what were to become standard elegiac tropes: *servitium amoris* ('the slavery of love'), *militia amoris* ('the battle of love') and *exclusus amator* ('the locked-out lover'). The fixation on a specific *puella* – Tibullus's Delia and Propertius's Cynthia – is also the inspiration for Ovid's Corinna. Both poets focus on women – not only as objects of desire – but as embodiments of female habits and concerns per se, which is particularly influential on the *Amores*.[28] In the adornment or cosmetic-themed poems of Ovid, principally

*Am.* 1.14, both Tibullus and Propertius's interest in matters pertaining to women is evident. Assuming the role of the *praeceptor amoris* in 1.8, ostensibly a homoerotic response to Marathus and his tryst with Pholoe, Tibullus explains his amatory credentials then proceeds to comment on the unappealing nature of ornate and artificial adornment (1.8.9–16), beginning with a couplet, 1.8.9–10:

> Quid tibi nunc molles prodest coluisse capillos
>     saepeque mutatas disposuisse comas?
>
> What good does it do now to have adorned soft locks
>     and to have styled your often-changed tresses?

Tibullus's message on the *cultus* of the elegiac *puella* is clear: she is most pleasing when unadorned (cf. Booth 1996; Damer 2014); of course, the lines are echoed in *Am.* 1.14.1. Following the lines on beautification, Tibullus employs what are to become by Ovid's time, standard themes of Latin elegy, such as a discourse against magic (1.8.17–26) and warnings against the ravages of old age (1.8.41–46).

In her study of the *Amores*, Morgan (1977: 2) problematizes the debt to Propertius, citing among other poems, *Am.*1.14: 'Just because both Propertius and Ovid wrote poems about dyeing the hair, does not ... mean that Ovid was directly copying Propertius.... It seems more likely that Ovid is repeating a cliché of the genre' (cf. also, Berman 1972; Zetzel 1996; Boyd 1997: 117–122). This statement provides a useful case study of *Am.* 1.14 and its interaction with Propertius (and Tibullus).

Morgan is both right and wrong. In *Am.* 1.14 Ovid directly imitates Propertius, and yet a preference for natural feminine beauty expressed in the same poem is *also* an elegiac cliché. Ovid's imitation of Propertius's 1.9.1 –

> Dicebam tibi venturos, irrisor, amores
> I was constantly saying, mocking one, that love would come

– is evident in *Am.* 1.14.1:

> Dicebam 'medicare tuos desiste capillos'
> I was constantly saying 'Desist from treating your locks'

Additionally, *Am.* 1.14.1 references both Propertius's 1.2.1 –

> Quid iuvat ornato procedere, vita, capillo?
> What use is it to come, my life, with locks adorned?

– and Tibullus 1.8.9–10 (quoted above). Yet the ultimate tone of *Am.* 1.14 is far from the earnest opprobrium of these poets. Verbal echoes may exist but Ovid's version is light with a decidedly parodic edge. His use of both Propertius and Tibullus shows the same hallmarks of his poetic responses to Virgil who is also referenced in the *Amores* (for an obvious example, cf. *Am.* 1.1 and *Aeneid* 1.1); flaunting imitation and clichés and producing elegies with 'a perverse kind of originality' (Zetzel 1996: 100).

Like the *Medicamina*, the *Amores* pays deference to the Alexandrians.[29] The preface makes this clear by mentioning that the second edition is slimmer[30] and by assuming a personified form that references Callimachus's chatty nautilus shell (*Epigram* 6 Pfeiffer 1953) and talking lock of hair (*Fragment* 110 Pfeiffer 1965).[31] The latter poem, known as the 'Lock of Berenice' and imitated by Catullus (66),[32] is worthy of a brief analysis here to demonstrate Ovid's innovative treatment of an Alexandrian original – and a Latin version – in *Am.* 1.14.

The inventiveness of Ovid's version is partly achieved by a carnivalesque reduction of this romantic tale. Queen Berenice II of Egypt is an archetypal heroine of antiquity, characterized by her wifely devotion to Ptolemy III Euergetes (reigned 246–222 BC) who, in turn, epitomized an ideal leader and husband. Berenice, who vowed to dedicate a lock of hair to ensure her husband's safety in his march against Syria, dutifully fulfilled her obligation on Euergetes' return, and her lock was committed to the gods (cf. Gutzwiller 1992). After the dedication to Aphrodite-Arsinoe in the temple at Zephyrium, the lock vanished, carried up to the heavens by Zephyrus on the command of the goddess, and became a new constellation. This well-known fantasy, intrinsically Alexandrian, with Theocritus also treating it (*Idyll* 17), and intrinsically neoteric, with Catullus's imitation (66), becomes parodic dynamite in Ovid's hands. Ovid combines the romance of Berenice's lock with the anti-cosmetic sentiments of Tibullus and Propertius to create an original discourse on the modern woman of the late-first century BC. Far from the dedicated spouse who is honoured by the goddess of love, Corinna is a poet's mistress whose locks fall out because she has over-treated them with dye and hot curling irons. The romantic story of a graceful, royal woman thus rematerializes in *Am.* 1.14 as an unromantic comedy of errors.

## Ars Amatoria

The first two Books of the *Ars* are feisty, at times incendiary, male-centred elegies with overtones of the sympotic songs of the Greek tradition. All manner of advice is given on the topic of controlling *amor* for the benefit of the individual male student with Ovid's overall dictum being that it should be approached like a career (on the latter, cf. Solodow 1977). To harness *amor* for the benefit of the *amator* one must learn the appropriate *artes* (*AA* 1.1-4). With an eye on the moral panopticon of the Augustan regime, Ovid makes it clear that the prescribed *artes* will ensure safe love-making and permitted secrecy while avoiding *crimen* or offence (*AA* 1.33-34). It failed, as we know, and along with the mysterious *error* (*carmen et error*, *Tr.* 2.207), resulted in Ovid's relegation to Tomis.[33]

While the first two Books of the collection are all about men, Ovid does foreshadow his next book and its female audience at *AA* 2.745-746:

> Ecce, rogant tenerae sibi idem praecepta puellae:
> vos eritis chartae proxima cura meae.

> Look, delicate girls are begging me to provide teaching:
> you will be my tablet's next concern.

Sharrock (1994) reads these lines as a carefully constructed revelation of an agenda that was present all along, namely that the *Ars* was always going to be about men *and* women, and Book Three was always part of the plan. This strategy, unveiled in the last two lines of Book Two, was intended to surprise the male readers of Books One and Two and was, adopting Sharrock's argument, cleverly concealed until then. While there are alternative views (cf. Henderson 2006 who suggests the surprise is not a surprise at all), Sharrock's thesis maintains a disjuncture between the sexes that is suitably Roman. It also underscores the distinctly male perspectives at play in the erotodidactic corpus overall: the reductive assumption that (all) contemporary women are concerned with enhancing their faces and preserving their looks; the preference for the well-presented woman over the one disinterested in attracting the male gaze; and the correlation between female adornment within the context of male precepts.

Turning to the authorial influences on the *Ars*, we see the reappearance of artistic ancestors already discussed in relation to other works. Therefore, in order to avoid repetition, the collection's erotodidactic nature is examined through the keyhole of sex manuals. We begin with Philaenis (*fl.* fourth century BC), author of an erotic handbook, of which only fragments remain (*Oxyrhynchus Papyri* 39: 2891 Lobel): part of a preface, a section on seduction (with a heading), a piece on flattery (without a heading) and a heading entitled 'On Kissing' (without a text).[34] The fragment from the preface introduces the author, explains that the book is for those who wish to be instructed with knowledge accrued from scientific enquiry, and specifies the toil entailed in the composition. On seduction, Philaenis advises a man to come to the object of desire in a dishevelled state to avoid appearing predatory. In the advice on flattery, a man is to compare his beloved to a goddess; if she is ugly she is told she is charming, and if she is old she is told she is like a young girl. The first piece of advice corresponds roughly to *Ars* 1.505–524 in respect to the expectation that a man should not be too fussy about his appearance, while the second is close to *AA* 2.657–666 on avoiding talk of a woman's flaws. It is likely that Philaenis discussed – or described – the best positions for sex, also at *Ars* 3.769–788, although Lobel maintains that the work must have been much broader than instructions on sexual positions – as the pieces mentioned above demonstrate – leading him to describe it as 'a systematic exposition of *ars amatoria*' (Lobel as per Tsantsanoglou 1973: 183). Taking Lobel's cue, therefore, allows one to posit that Philaenis may well have covered all of the bases of *Ars* Book Three (cf. Parker 1992). In addition to Philaenis, Ovid would have also had access to other handbooks, such as the didactic poetry of Elephantis (*fl.* first century BC) on sex and also medicine, a part of which, on abortifacients, is summarized by Pliny (28.81),[35] and another part, on cosmetics, is referenced by Galen (12.416 Kühn 1826).

In addition to such manuals, Myerowitz argues that Ovid was also most likely inspired by erotic *tabellae* (lit. 'small paintings') similar to the scenes from the House of the Vettii in Pompeii. For support, Myerowitz (1992: 156n3) notes the specific references to *tabellae* by Propertius, Pliny, Suetonius,

Plutarch, Athenaeus, the Priapea and *AA* 2.679–680 in which Ovid mentions that women are adept in assuming novel positions that went far beyond erotic paintings. While the intention(s) behind the inclusion of such decorative works in private homes is open to debate, there may well have been a didactic element to them. Myerowitz (1992: 148) notes Brendel's discussion of the paintings as originally sourced from illustrated handbooks and thereby serving a specifically didactic purpose – as well as a titillating one. Interestingly, in *Tr.* 2.521–528 Ovid implies that Augustus owned a *tabella* on which were depicted scenes of heroic or mythological figures demonstrating various sexual positions.

## *Remedia Amoris*

Some scholars (Küppers 1981; Wildberger 1998; Rimell 2006) have suggested that the *Remedia* may be read as part four of the *Ars*, which consequently makes a quadrilateral series like Virgil's *Georgics*. Indeed, the poem is regularly in dialogue with the *Ars*, maintaining the emphases on *artes*, *amor* and *puellae*. But, as Rosati (2006) has discussed, the *Remedia* also connects with the *Amores*, beginning, like it does, with Amor. As Ovid was led to elegy by Amor in the *Amores*, he finds the god present once more as he composes the *Remedia*, except this time, Amor is alert to a war about to be waged against him (*l*.2). Ovid manages to persuade Amor, however, that the young men (*iuvenes*) sick with his wounds also need instruction; thus, at *ll*.39–40, the god acquiesces:

> Haec ego; movit Amor gemmatas aureus alas,
>   et mihi 'propositum perfice' dixit 'opus.'

> Thus spoke I; golden Amor moved his bejewelled wings,
>   and to me 'finish the proposed work' he said.

Not surprising, Ovid is indifferent to, and at times negative towards, *cultus* in the *Remedia*. Like the women he seeks to undo, the benefits and charms of *cultus* are minimized and sometimes scorned. Ovid ceases to wax lyrical on the evolutionary wonders of *cultus*; unlike the *Medicamina* and *Ars* Book Three, he does not marvel at the gifts of agriculture, but instead observes that the earth still produces noxious plants as well as healing herbs and the nettle still grows next to the rose (*ll*.45–46). This is an inspired metaphor to foreshadow the woman at her toilette at *ll*.343–356 who, as it turns out, is more nettle than rose, and more inclined to dip into noxious substances for her beautification rather than the pleasant herbs and sweet ingredients of the *Medicamina*.

As we read Ovid's remedies, it soon becomes clear that he has spent a good deal of time contemplating satire and perhaps, according to Rosati (2006), even magical treatises. As with the section on the sources of imitation in the *Ars*, which acknowledged standard works but then moved on to discuss additional ones, this analysis of the generic and poetic inspirations for the *Remedia* does the same, and focuses on satire.

Satire is present in other works by Ovid but usually not to the same degree as the *Remedia*, which is not surprising considering its theme. With its aim to end desire and redirect its energies elsewhere, there is a particular need for the unleashing of the satirist's *stilus*. The object of desire requires the poet's skills in the areas of *reductio ad absurdum* and *reductio ad obscenam*. Ovid himself admits the use of the iambic metre is the most appropriate means, poetically, of driving off unwanted lovers and beckons it at *ll*.377–378, thereby invoking the satirists' links to the Greek iambic tradition of Archilochus, Semonides and Hipponax, and their poetry of vituperation. So too, Horace's *Satires* I and II (36–35 BC and 29–25 BC) as well as the often dark and foreboding elegies of the *Epodes* (32–30 BC), are present as important successors to the Greek tradition and important precursors to the *Remedia*.

The application of the satirist's misogyny – be it an affectation or something more – is important to this study because of its traditional use of motifs oppositional to much of the imagery of Ovid's evocations of feminine *cultus*. Rhetorically speaking, the combative voice of the satirist is needed in the *Remedia* and manifests itself in a passage selected herein, namely *ll*.343–356 on the anti-cosmetic tradition. It surfaces with far more vigour in *ll*.437–440 in Ovid's reluctant suggestion – immediately retracted – to watch the *puella* performing *obscena* (the adjective used as a substantive plural, denoting actions that are 'ill-omened' or 'obscene'; here meaning the bodily functions of defecation / urination). The focus on the woman's body as excessively moist, be it with mucky, greasy, malodorous creams (*ll*.351–356) or the moisture of bodily fluids expelled, creates an image of an abject *puella* far removed from the elegiac beloved.[36]

Such female-centred tropes of cruel observation and exaggeration come some thirty years after Horace's major works of satire and iambic, and the debt is evident. In *Epode* 12.1–20, Horace revels in a gross description of an old prostitute, evoking images of the stench of poor hygiene, hairy armpits (possibly hiding a goat), her oily and unstable foundation and her rouge of 'crocodile' shit (*stercus*). He extends the vituperation by evoking memories of her genitals, which are pungent and shrivelled, which foreshadows Ovid's anecdotal advice concerning a close-up of a woman's 'obscene parts' (*obscenae partes*) and an inspection of the 'shameful marks' (*signa pudenda*) she leaves on a 'filthy bed' (*inmundus torus*), as effective means of killing desire (*Rem.* 429–432).

Reminiscent of the fragment of the *Isostasion* in which the physical faults of prostitutes are alleviated with artificial interventions, Ovid suggests that an effective cure for *amor* is to fixate on a woman's flaws (*Rem.* 325–342). This inversion of the bitter realism and misogyny of New Comedy not only suggests Ovid's familiarity with Alexis's play and its genre per se, but also his skills in accentuating the, at times, blurred lines between comedy and satire for biting effect. Perhaps more importantly, such nasty passages, which often trouble scholars because of the intratextual contradictions of other works within the Ovidian oeuvre, are revealed as nothing more than rhetorical devices to suit a given *topos*. Ovid goes where his Muse takes him.

# Notes

1 There is an extensive history of beautification procedures prior to the age of Ovid. The first accounts of corrective surgery for facial defects are preserved in the *Edwin Smith Papyrus* (*c.* 3000 BC), cf. Rinzler (2009: 150ff.). In India by *c.* 800 BC, reconstructive surgery was being practised, with various techniques recorded in the Sanskrit text, the *Sushruta Samhita* (*c.* sixth century BC), cf. Bhishagratna (1907). For a concise history of elective plastic surgery in antiquity, cf. Marmelzat (1987) and, on cosmeceuticals and cosmetics in the ancient world, cf. Blanco-Dávila (2000).

2  Xenophon employs several key cosmetic terms in Greek. Ischomachus's wife uses *psimythion* ('white lead') to lighten her skin (cf. p. 70) and *egkhousa* ('alkanet'), which has a root that produces a red dye for rouge. Ischomachus, in his hypothetical depiction of himself after having applied cosmetics, mentions *miltos* or red ochre for his cheeks and also *andreikelos*, a flesh-coloured pigment.

3  On feminine adornment, including jewellery, cosmeceuticals and cosmetics in Juvenal, cf. Watson (2007), and also Watson and Watson (2014: 223–228).

4  On *pudicitia*, cf. Langlands (2006).

5  Probably not the famous Egyptian queen; cf. Parker (2012: 379).

6  The references to Balsdon and Seneca are from Stewart (2007: 54). On the possibility that women's baths also catered for beauty treatments, Stewart comments: 'Interestingly, tools believed to be surgical instruments have been found at bath complexes. The presence of these items may suggest that minor surgical operations, at least, may have been carried out on the premises.... However, cosmetic utensils including long-handled spoons (*ligulae*), spatulas and palettes do resemble surgical tools ... It is possible that the bath administration may have profited from the sale of cosmetics and perfumes on their premises, as they did from other services offered to clients including catering and massage. No doubt individual women attending the baths may have reapplied their make-up and scent once they had bathed but finding concrete evidence for the sale or application of cosmetics and perfumes as a service provided for customers needs much more investigation.'

7  Cf. Fagan (1999: 85–103). Not surprisingly, there were critics of bathing, particularly when it came to frequent bathing; cf. Toner (1995: 53–64). Toner notes those opponents of such activities who saw attention to bodily cleanliness – particularly among men – as symptomatic of increasing femininity among Roman men and as a sign of general moral decline.

8  This mirror is without a handle and designed to fit comfortably in the palm. For a detailed discussion of the artefact, cf. Milleker (1998).

9  This is borne out by Shumka (2008: 173) in her work on representations of the *mundus muliebris* on funerary monuments. Of particular note is her discussion of the goodly matron who also spent time on her appearance in a modest way: 'Depending upon time, finances, or desire, a woman might turn her attention to adornment, apparel, complexion management, hair care and styling, or any combination of these endeavours. If performed conscientiously, this art produced an elegant appearance that publicly and privately asserted her gender identity.'

10  Throughout, *munditia* is translated as 'simple elegance' to best encapsulate Ovid's use of the term (cf. Watson 2002: 144).

11 Cf. Watson (1982) for discussion of the distinctions in Ovid's approaches to beautification and *ars* in the *Medicamina* and *Ars* Book Three. Watson argues that, while the *Medicamina* presents a *praeceptor* who adopts a traditional approach to *cultus* in terms of his casual recommendations of, at times, luxury items, the *Ars* depicts him as a mixture of *lena* ('procuress') and *pauper poeta* ('impoverished poet'). While the former requires an expensively adorned girl to attract wealthy clients, the latter avoids recommending costly items because they place financial burdens on poor boyfriends. The key is artistry, not extravagance.

12 On the motif of the *custos* ('guard') in *AA* 3.611–658, cf. Gibson (2003: 334–349).

13 On the irreversible and ever-increasing importation of luxury items during the Augustan age (and its representation in poetry), cf. Griffin (1976). On Ovidian women, *cultus* and empire, cf. also Bowditch (2012), especially: 'Ovid's elegiac-didactic poetry, in particular, suggests the favourable conditions to international commerce that came about with the *Pax Augusta*. The *Medicamina Faciei Femineae*, a handbook devoted to cosmetics, openly advertises the advantages of *imperium sine fine* for improving female appearance.' (Ibid. 128).

14 He reiterates the message of *AA* 1.31–34 as a means of self-defence in the exile poems; cf., for example, *Tr.* 2.212, 346 and *Ep.* 3.3.51–52.

15 On the reintroduction or promotion of traditional attire, cf. Zanker (1990: 162–166). Cf. also, Sebesta (1997), particularly on a statue of Livia, wife of Augustus, in which she is depicted wearing not only the *stola* and *vittae* but has her *palla* ('long robe' or 'mantle') covering her head (Ibid. 56); cf. National Archaeological Museum, Naples, Inv. Neg. Rom. 76.1157. It is important to note that extant ancient sources do not indicate that Augustus legislated on women's attire. For further discussion, cf. Watson and Watson (2014: 220).

16 The intricacies of the law remain difficult to interpret regarding the exact classes of women included in it and those exempt from it; cf. McGinn (1991). As the law specified the *mater familias*, 'whether she was married or not' (335n3), as the female category 'potentially liable to its penalties', it seems plausible, as McGinn argues, that only prostitutes and procuresses were exempt from the *lex Iulia*. In line with McGinn's interpretation, the law would have included freedwomen under its jurisdiction, which in turn problematizes the meaning of the term *matrona* ('married woman', 'wife', 'mother') within the traditional context of the Roman elite. On this point, cf. Veyne (1998: 74): 'How could former slaves be considered true matrons when they had not been raised and protected as virgins in order to become wives ...?' Ovid's narrow definition of who exactly is a *matronae* at *AA.* 1.31–34 may therefore be a sly allusion to the uncertainty concerning members of this class within the confines of the *lex Iulia*.

17 Other common and often stable terms also become unclear and contested in the erotodidactic texts, particularly the *Ars*; cf. Watson (2002: 156) on words such as *vir* and *puella*. Cf. also Davis (1999: 445) on *Am.* 2.12.1–4 and the reference to Corinna's *vir* (*l*.3), which, in this context is ambiguous – does the poet mean her husband or her lover? 'We cannot tell.'

18 The *Medicamina* is usually dated to c. 2 BC, based in part on *AA* 3.205, which leads scholars such as Rosati (1985: 42–43) to suggest a date between *AA* Books One and Two (2 BC) and *AA* Book Three (AD 2). Lenz (1965: 81) posits that *AA* Books 1 and 2 were composed simultaneously with the *Medicamina*, while Hollis (1977: xii) dates the work somewhat earlier, arguing that it was a 'trial run' for the *Ars Amatoria*. Neither Lenz nor Hollis diverge radically from Rosati.

19 Toohey (2013: 161) draws attention to the inclusion of the second person singular – 'you' – in the second half of the poem; contra Watson (2001: 459n9).

20 Cf., for example, Scene 8 from the fresco in the Villa of the Mysteries at Pompeii and 'Venus at her Toilet' from Thuburbo-Majus (Bardo Museum, Tunis).

21 Transgressing the boundaries of privacy is a poetic conceit favoured by Ovid, as attested by his penchant for 'reading' people's mail in the *Heroides* and for revealing the secrets of others (cf. the discussion of Corinna's abortion in *Am.* 2.13 and 2.14). Often the sneak, he also eavesdrops (*Am.* 1.8.21ff.) and spies (*Am.* 2.5.13ff.).

22 Cf. Fränkel (1945: 63): 'From this work only fifty couplets have survived, and we have probably no reason to regret the loss of the rest.'

23 In addition to the scholarship mentioned above, other important studies on the *Medicamina* include the early work by Kunz (1881); studies by Leary (1988a, 1988b, 1990); Nikolaidis (1994); García (1995); and Cioccoloni (2006). The text is also included to varying degrees in research on Roman cosmetics; cf. Saiko (2005); Stewart (2007); and Olson (2008a, 2008b, 2009).

24 Further on Callimachean echoes in *Am.* 3.1 and in the collection per se, cf., McKeown (1987: 1: 32–62); Acosta-Hughes (2009: 250). The echoes of *Iambus* 4 as discussed by Acosta-Hughes may have been an additional acknowledgement of the metrical debt to Callimachus.

25 On the influence of Nicander on the *Medicamina*, cf. Rosati (1985: 47). On Nicander's work on metamorphoses, *Heteroeoumena* (*The Book of Changed Things*), preserved in a prose summary by Antoninus Liberalis, and Ovid's *Metamorphoses*, cf. Griffin (1981 and 1991). Aratus's influence is also important, with a non-extant poem in hexameter titled the *Aratea*, almost certainly inspired by Aratus's *Phaenomena*.

26 Theophrastus refers to the plant as the Persian apple (*mēlon*). On the relevant passage of Theophrastus and the use and adaptation of it by Virgil, cf. Thomas

(1987: 236). Thomas (Ibid. 253–260) provides further and more extensive analyses of Virgil's direct use of Theophrastus in the *Georgics* and cites Jahn and also Mitsdörffer. In addition to Theophrastus, the *Georgics* also reflects the influences of Aratus and Nicander; cf. Gale (2000).

27 *Georgics* 2.109–135 is preceded by a digression on the misuse of botanical properties by stepmothers, against which the citron offers an antidote (2.126–130).* Virgil returns to the trope of plants and stepmothers at *Georgics* 3.282–283 in his description of the magical ingredient, *hippomanes* (cf. p. 56). Similarly, Ovid writes of the potentially dangerous uses of herbs at *Med. ll.*35–38, warning his female audience against meddling in botanical potions, including the infamous ingredient, *hippomanes,* for magical purposes (cf. also *Am.* 1.14.39–40). The powers of nature are treated with respect by both poets and their concern is that cultivation be confined to positive activities and outcomes.

* *Georgics* 2.129 is regarded by some as an interpolation; cf. Thomas (1988: 178); for a detailed discussion, cf. Watson (1993).

28 The *Tristia* provides the most informative accounts of Ovid's interaction with the elegies of Tibullus and Propertius. Cf., for example, *Tr.* 2.447–448, on Ovid's analysis of the works of both poets and their influence on his own oeuvre. In an excellent study of this passage and its detailed homage to several of Tibullus's works, cf. James (2003: 159–160).

29 The choice of the elegiac metre over the hexameter for a didactic work such as the *Medicamina* references Callimachus's *Aetia*; likewise, if, as discussed above, the *Medicamina* was relatively compact in size, it pays heed to the Alexandrian preference for brevity. The scholarship on Alexandrian influences on Ovid is immense; for some examples, cf. Miller (1983); Boyd (1997); Hunter (2006); Lightfoot (2009); Acosta-Hughes (2009); Keith (2011).

30 Cf. Barchiesi (1988: 102–103) for the suggestion that perhaps the first edition was nothing more than a poetic ploy to provide a witty introduction to the collection; cf. also Cameron (1968); Boyd (1997). Cf. Jansen (2012) for a discussion of the suggestion.

31 Cf. also Catullus 67 on the house door and Propertius 1.16 on the same. Further on talking prefatory poems in Callimachus, cf. McKeown (1989: 2: 2); for Alexandrian influences on the elegiac precursors to Ovid – a most exhausting topic – cf. Lightfoot (2009); Acosta-Hughes (2009); on Catullus in particular, cf. Wheeler (1934); Ross (1969); Du Quesnay (2012); Nelis (2012). On the significance of Alexandrian influences on neoteric poets and their successors per se as well as technical approaches to *imitatio,* cf. Hinds (1998).

32 On the possibility of the allusion, cf. McKeown (1989: 2: 365); also Zetzel (1996: 77). Catullus's influence on Ovid is extensive and has only been referenced briefly herein; for a detailed study, cf. Wray (2009: 252–264).
33 Ovid's *relegatio* is an exhaustive scholarly topic, and cannot be dealt with in detail. For some examples of influential scholarship, cf. Norwood (1963); Green (1982); Holleman (1971); Goold (1983); Williams (1994); McGowan (2009). For the *relegatio* as poetic fantasy, cf. Fitton Brown (1985); Hejduk (2014: 34–40). For a concise survey of the topic, cf. Claassen (2008).
34 Philaenis was traditionally thought to have been a courtesan, although modern scholars tend to argue that the name is a pseudonym to disguise a male author. Cf. Tsantsanoglou (1973); cf. in particular the discussion of ancient disputes concerning her identity (Ibid.: 185–186). The readings adopted are based on the text as emended by Parker (1992) and Parker (1989).
35 In the same section, Pliny mentions the work of Lais (unknown) on abortifacients. Elephantis is also mentioned by Martial (12.43.4) as the author of a sex manual in verse and referred to by Suetonius (*Tiberius* 43.2) as a favourite of Tiberius.
36 I owe this reading to the work of Brunelle (2005), whose study is an excellent, persuasive interpretation of the *Remedia* from the perspective of the genre of satire.

# 1

## *Medicamina Faciei Femineae*

### Latin text

Discite quae faciem commendet cura, puellae,
  et quo sit vobis forma tuenda modo.

Cultus humum sterilem Cerealia pendere iussit
  munera, mordaces interiere rubi.
Cultus et in pomis sucos emendat acerbos, 5
  fissaque adoptivas accipit arbor opes.
Culta placent. Auro sublimia tecta linuntur,
  nigra sub imposito marmore terra latet.
Vellera saepe eadem Tyrio medicantur aeno;
  sectile deliciis India praebet ebur. 10

Forsitan antiquae Tatio sub rege Sabinae
  maluerint quam se rura paterna coli,
cum matrona premens altum rubicunda sedile
  assiduo durum pollice nebat opus,
ipsaque claudebat quos filia paverat agnos, 15
  ipsa dabat virgas caesaque ligna foco.

At vestrae matres teneras peperere puellas:
  vultis inaurata corpora veste tegi,
vultis odoratos positu variare capillos,
  conspicuam gemmis vultis habere manum; 20
induitis collo lapides Oriente petitos
  et quantos onus est aure tulisse duos.
Nec tamen indignum: sit vobis cura placendi,

    cum comptos habeant saecula nostra viros:
feminea vestri poliuntur lege mariti                            25
    et vix ad cultus nupta quod addat habet.

†Pro se quaeque parent et quos venerentur amores,
    refert. Munditia crimina nulla merent.†
Rure latent finguntque comas, licet arduus illas
    celet Athos, cultas altus habebit Athos.                   30
Est etiam placuisse sibi quaecumque voluptas:
    virginibus cordi grataque forma sua est.
Laudatas homini volucris Iunonia pennas
    explicat et forma muta superbit avis.

Sic potius nos urget amor quam fortibus herbis,          35
    quas maga terribili subsecat arte manus.
Nec vos graminibus nec mixto credite suco,
    nec temptate nocens virus amantis equae.
Nec mediae Marsis finduntur cantibus angues,
    nec redit in fontes unda supina suos.                     40
Et quamvis aliquis Temesaea removerit aera,
    numquam Luna suis excutietur equis.

Prima sit in vobis morum tutela, puellae:
    ingenio facies conciliante placet.
Certus amor morum est: formam populabitur aetas,     45
    et placitus rugis vultus aratus erit;
tempus erit quo vos speculum vidisse pigebit
    et veniet rugis altera causa dolor.
Sufficit et longum probitas perdurat in aevum,
    perque suos annos hinc bene pendet amor.               50

Discite, cum teneros somnus dimiserit artus,
    candida quo possint ora nitere modo.

Hordea, quae Libyci ratibus misere coloni,
    exue de palea tegminibusque suis:
par ervi mensura decem madefiat ab ovis                    55

sed cumulent libras hordea nuda duas.
Haec, ubi ventosas fuerint siccata per auras,
    lenta iube scabra frangat asella mola.
Et quae prima cadent vivaci cornua cervo
    contere – in haec solidi sexta fac assis eat.     60
Iamque ubi pulvereae fuerint confusa farinae,
    protinus innumeris omnia cerne cavis;
adice narcissi bis sex sine cortice bulbos
    (strenua quos puro marmore dextra terat)
sextantemque trahat gummi cum semine Tusco;     65
    huc novies tanto plus tibi mellis eat.
Quaecumque afficiet tali medicamine vultum,
    fulgebit speculo levior illa suo.

Nec tu pallentes dubita torrere lupinos,
    et simul inflantes corpora frige fabas:     70
utraque sex habeant aequo discrimine libras,
    utraque da pigris comminuenda molis.
Nec cerussa tibi nec nitri spuma rubentis
    desit et Illyrica quae venit iris humo:
da validis iuvenum pariter subigenda lacertis     75
    (sed iustum tritis uncia pondus erit).

Addita de querulo volucrum medicamina nido
    ore fugant maculas; alcyonea vocant.
Pondere, si quaeris quo sim contentus in illis,
    quod trahit in partes uncia secta duas.     80
Ut coeant apteque lini per corpora possint,
    adice de flavis Attica mella favis.

Quamvis tura deos irataque numina placent,
    non tamen accensis omnia danda focis.
Tus ubi miscueris radenti tubera nitro,     85
    ponderibus iustis fac sit utrimque triens.
Parte minus quarta dereptum cortice gummi,
    et modicum e myrrhis pinguibus adde cubum.

Haec, ubi contrieris, per densa foramina cerne;
    pulvis ab infuso melle premendus erit.                                              90

Profuit et marathos bene olentibus addere myrris –
    quinque trahant marathi scripula, myrra novem –
arentisque rosae quantum manus una prehendat,
    cumque Ammoniaco mascula tura sale.
Hordea quem faciunt, illis affunde cremorem                       95
    (aequent expensas cum sale tura rosas).
Tempore sint parvo molli licet illita vultu,
    haerebit toto nullus in ore color.

Vidi quae gelida madefacta papavera lympha
    contereret teneris illineretque genis.                                              100

*   *   *   *   *   *   *   *

## Translation

Learn what treatment may enhance your face, girls,
    and the means by which you must preserve your looks.
Cultivation commanded the barren earth to render Ceres'
    'gifts', the stinging brambles, to perish.
Cultivation removes bitterness from the juice of fruits,                5
    and the grafted tree receives acquired wealth.
Cultivations give pleasure. Soaring halls are lined with gold,
    the black earth lies hid beneath superimposed marble.
The same fleeces are dipped often in a Tyrian cauldron;
    India proffers carved ivory for ornamentations.                    10

Perhaps, under Tatius' reign, the ancient Sabine women would
    have preferred their fathers' farms be cultivated rather than themselves,
while the ruddy-cheeked matron, sitting on her high chair,
    spun her laborious task with constantly-moving thumb,

and she herself enclosed the lambs her daughter had pastured, 15
   and herself put kindling and hewn logs on the hearth.

But *your* mothers gave birth to tender girls:
   you want your bodies swathed in gold-embroidered garments,
you want to variegate your scented locks by means of styling,
   you want to have your hands admired for their precious stones; 20
you adorn your neck with gems sourced from the East,
   so large that it is a burden to bear two of them on the ear.
But this is not unworthy behaviour: you must be anxious to please,
   since our age possesses well-groomed men.
Your husbands smooth their skin in line with the law of women 25
   so that even a wife could scarcely add anything to their cultivation.

†Pro se quaeque parent et quos venerentur amores,
   refert. Munditia crimina nulla meret.†
Women bury themselves in the countryside and yet arrange their tresses,
   though rugged Athos conceal them, lofty Athos will have cultivated
      women. 30
There is even a certain kind of delight in pleasing oneself:
   for young girls dear to their heart is their beauty.
The bird of Juno unfurls feathers, praiseworthy in the eyes of mankind,
   and in silence the bird exults in its beauty.

Thus it is more likely that passion drives us rather than powerful herbs, 35
   which the sorceress' hand plucks with a frightful art.
Do not place your trust in grasses or a mix of juices,
   try not the baneful venom of a mare on heat.
Snakes are not split down the middle by Marsian spells,
   the wave is not reversed and returned to its own source. 40
And though someone may have set aside Temesaean bronze,
   the Moon will never be shaken from her chariot.

First and foremost, girls, should be the protection of your moral fibre:
   overall appearance gives pleasure when it recommends character.
Love of good character is assured: age will ravage beauty, 45
   and, features once pleasing, will be ploughed by wrinkles;

there will be a time when it will displease you to look in a mirror
    and grief will become another cause of wrinkles.
Probity is the bedrock and it endures throughout a lengthy lifetime,
    and it is from it that love securely depends.   50

Learn, when sleep has released your tender limbs,
    how your face could shine radiantly.

Strip the barley, which farmers from Libya have sent by ship,
    of its husks and coverings:
an equal measure of bitter vetch is soaked in ten eggs:   55
    but the stripped barley should amount to two *librae*.
Once dried by gusty breezes, have these
    crushed on a rough millstone by a slow she-ass.
Grind into this the first horns that fall from a long-lived stag –
    see that a sixth of a whole *as* goes in.   60
Next, having mixed this into the pounded meal, you must
    immediately sift every last granule through closely-meshed strainers;
add twelve narcissus bulbs minus the rind
    (which a vigorous right-hand should grind on clean marble)
and let gum along with Tuscan seed weigh one-sixth of an *as*;   65
    into it let there go nine times as much honey.
Any woman who applies this treatment to her face,
    will gleam more smoothly than her own mirror.

Nor must you hesitate to roast pale lupin-seeds,
    and at the same time to fry beans that make the body swell:   70
and let each of these have six *librae* in equal measure,
    and give each to the slow-moving millstone to be thoroughly refined.
Let neither white lead nor the scum of ruddy natron be lacking
    to you as well as the iris that comes from the soil of Illyricum:
give them all together to be pounded by the strong arms of young men,   75
    but the correct weight, once ground, will be an *uncia*.

Additional treatments taken from the querulous nest of birds
    put to flight blotches from the face; they call it *alcyonea*.

If you were to ask about a weight that would satisfy me, concerning these
    it is that which an *uncia*, divided into two portions, weighs.     80
That they may combine and be smeared easily over the body,
    add Attic honey from golden honeycombs.

Although frankincense can placate the gods and angry divine powers,
    not all, however, must be surrendered to burning hearths.
When you have mixed frankincense with the natron that smooths swellings,   85
    ensure there is a third of a *libra* from each in exact weighted portions.
To a cube of gum stripped of its rind less a quarter,
    also add a small cube of thick myrrh.
When you have ground these, sift through close-packed strainers;
    the powder will need to be compacted by an infusion of honey.     90

It is profitable also to mix well fennel with sweet smelling myrrh –
    the fennel weighing five *scripula*, the myrrh nine –
and as much as one hand can hold of dried rose-petals,
    and the finest frankincense with salt of Ammon.
Infuse these with the thick juice that barley makes     95
    (the frankincense should equal the weight of the rose petals and the salt).
Although these ingredients be smeared on your soft features
    only for a brief time, no colour will cling to the entire face.

I have seen one who crumbled poppies made moist by chilled
    water and smeared them on her tender cheeks.     100

        \*    \*    \*    \*    \*    \*    \*    \*

# Commentary

## Lines 1–2 – Opening couplet

The opening couplet introduces several key words:

    (i) *discite* ('learn'). The dramatic imperative, choice of verb, and placement immediately introduce the poem as didactic and Ovid as the *praeceptor amoris* or, more applicable in this case, the *praeceptor cultus* ('teacher of cultivation'). It is repeated at *l*.51 (cf. p. 138 for editors who read *dic age*).

(ii) *cura* ('treatment'); also 'taking good care' and 'application'. The word also means 'anxiety', 'concern' and 'care'. It is repeated at *l*.23, where the context requires the translation 'concern'; cf. also *AA* 3.105 where it is translated as 'care'.

(iii) *puellae* ('girls'); recurring at *l*.17 and *l*.43. This is the standard word used to designate the female object of the elegist's desire. Here its generality reinforces the egalitarian nature of Ovid's intended audience; the *Medicamina* is for all girls, because it has something to offer all of them. On surveys of the term *puella*, cf. Miller (2013); also Watson (1983).

(iv) *facies* ('appearance', 'form', 'beauty'). This is a comprehensive term that denotes one's overall shape or appearance, one's figure, one's face; cf. also *AA* 3.105 (twice, where it is translated as 'beauty'); *l*.137 ('face'); *l*.210 ('appearance').

(v) *forma* ('looks', 'beauty', 'appearance'). *forma* may denote beauty per se, but perhaps not in the first instance (*l*.2), as Ovid is concerned with a general female audience, and clearly one including women requiring assistance with beautification (cf. *Ars* 3.255–256). In other words, if his audience all looked like Venus (or Corinna on a good day) there would be no need for this work. As he says in *AA* 3.261: *rara tamen menda facies caret* ('Rare nevertheless is the face that lacks blemishes'). *forma* appears four times in the text, translated as 'looks' in the first instance, and as 'beauty' in the other lines: the beauty of young girls, the beauty of the peacock and the effect of wrinkles on beauty; cf. also *AA* 3.103 (twice), *ll*.134, 205, 217, 234 (translated as both 'looks' and 'beauty' depending on context); *AA* 1.509 ('appearance').

## Lines 3–10 – *cultus*

*cultus* ('cultivation') opens *l*.3, to emphasize it as the theme of the work. It is repeated at *l*.5 and *l*.26 ('cultivation'); the cognate *culta* in the plural is used in *l*.7 (lit. 'the products of cultivation'). The passive infinitive *coli* is rendered 'to be cultivated' at *l*.12 and the participle *cultae* as 'cultivated' at *l*.30. Cf. also *AA* 3.101 (twice), *ll*.102, 107, 127, 225.

The reference to Ceres initiates a series of images pertaining to cultivated nature. Cultivation causes 'stinging brambles to perish', removes the 'bitterness from the juice of fruits' and bestows the skill of grafting. In each example, nature has been improved upon by *cultus*; on the theme of *cultus* in this agricultural context and the links to the *Georgics*, cf. pp. 25–27; cf. also

Watson (2001: 457, 460) and Cioccoloni (2006: 99n10, 103). The imagery of *ll.*3–6 establishes a subtle connection to the overall theme of the work: like the unpleasant brambles, the bitter taste of juices and the grafted fruit trees, women are also improved upon by *cultus*; cf. Richlin (1995: 187–188) and Rimell (2005: 197) for feminist readings.

From *cultus* in a more artificial context, namely monumental architecture (*ll.*7–8), Ovid turns to examples appealing to women (*ll.*9–10). Firstly he refers to the rich purple-red dye obtained from the *Murex* (a family of sea snail), which was a luxury item from Tyre (a major city in Phoenicia). The process of achieving the colour was exceptionally labour-intensive; thousands of snails were required for one garment, which needed to be dyed repeatedly in order to obtain a rich colour that was fade-resistant. The verb employed to describe the process of dyeing is *medicare* (lit. 'to medicate' or 'to heal') and translated at *l.*9 as 'treated'; Ovid also uses the term at *Am.* 1.14.1 to describe the process of dyeing hair (pp. 87–88). Olson (2008a: 119n5) notes that 'Purple was the status color *par excellence*' and discusses (2008a: 12) its ambivalent reception by men as a colour of choice for women: 'Although women had a wide range of hues for their clothing, some authors did not consider purple seemly for women, probably because of the strong status implications involved'. Olson cites Plautus's comedy, *The Haunted House l.*289 as an early example of male disapproval of purple-clad women and Suetonius's *Caesar* 43 on Caesar's ban on wearing purple, presumably by both sexes, as part of his laws against extravagance (with some strictly defined exceptions). Olson (2008a: 12) rightly suggests that 'Caesar's restrictions on purple ... assumed women wore the color often', although the colour symbolized excessive luxury whether adopted by either sex. Further on purple, cf. Reinhold (1970).

The second example of luxurious cultivation is Indian ivory (*ebur*). Like Tyrian dye, ivory was a highly prized commodity in antiquity, as St. Clair (2003: 7) discusses: 'Whereas bone was cheap and readily available, ivory was a rare and valuable commodity and, even in times of plenty, a potent symbol of prestige. In the form of tusks, intricately fashioned works of art, or even on the hoof, ivory was hoarded, paraded, exhibited, and even burned as a sign of wealth and status'. While elite women wore ivory hairpins, rings and bangles, Ovid evokes a plethora of luxury items with the word *deliciae* (translated at *l.*10 as 'ornamentations'), suggesting all kinds of delightful pleasures (Rimell's *objets d'art* is a deft translation; cf. Rimell 2006: 45). *deliciae* is often found in Latin erotic elegy where it usually equates to 'darling' or 'delight', though it also means 'pet'; cf., for example, Catullus on Lesbia's bird, with a double-entendre on the meanings of 'darling' and 'pet' (2.1 and 3.4); on one who brings delight (6.1); on acts of delight between lovers (45.24 and 74.2).

## Lines 11–16 – Women of the past

The poet's interest in the Sabine women is well attested in his oeuvre. Unlike the more sexualized and provocative version of the legend in *AA* 1.101–134, his concern here is to represent the women as the epitome of old-fashioned, upright behaviour. They are hardworking in the household and render much assistance around the farm and thus epitomize womanly and wifely virtues, especially piety and chastity. Nevertheless, the tone is gently mocking – achieved via a painterly scene of earnest, earthy women eschewing *cultus* in the Ovidian sense. Living during the reign of the Sabine king, Titus Tatius, a contemporary of Romulus, they understand *cultus* only in relation to rusticity; note the pun on *coli* ('to be cultivated') at *l*.12 in the context of the land being cultivated as opposed to the cultivation of the female body. Thus, rather than concerning herself with ornate clothing and beauty treatments, an austere Sabine *matrona* with ruddy (*rubicunda*) cheeks sits on her high chair and spins yarn; cf. Lovén (1998). As a pale or 'peaches and cream' complexion was valued in females, these Sabine women, sunburned in tending to their farms, show a regrettable (to Ovid) *insouciance* as to their appearance; cf. Watson (2003: 109) on *Epode* 2.41–42 and Horace's image of a farmer's sunburned wife. For sources on the Sabines, cf. Livy 1.10–14; Propertius 2.32; Tacitus *Annals* 1.54 and *History* 2.95; Plutarch *Romulus* 19–24. For Ovid, cf. *Am.* 1.8.39–40, 2.4.15–16, 2.12.21–24, 3.8.61 (where the *Sabinae* are essentially a stock motif for frigidity). On the Sabine women in Ovid's collected works, cf. Sharrock (2006); Labate (2006); further on Ovid, Rome's rustic past and *cultus*, cf. Watson (1982).

## Lines 17–26 – Women of the present

The Sabine story prompts Ovid to consider the daughters and mothers of his own era – females who are very different to their ancestors. He marks the transition from one age to the next by the conjunction *at* ('but'), which emphasizes the contrast between the women. Unlike the hardworking Sabine girl, the girls of Ovid's time will not end up with unattractive complexions through physical labour and neglected skin.

Ovid employs two examples of distinctly elegiac language in the couplets dealing with the women of the early imperial age: the women, designated as *puellae*, are described as *tenerae* ('tender', 'delicate', 'soft'); cf. Catullus 35.1; Ovid *AA* 3.333; *Rem. l.*757. The vocabulary evokes an image of the women as gentle, genteel, incapable of hard work and, as revealed in the lines that follow, lovers of luxury. That these *puellae* are the products of their mothers and their upbringing is suggested at *l.*17: *at vestrae matres teneras peperere puellas* ('But your mothers gave birth to tender girls'). Love of *cultus* is now, it seems, something one inherits, something a mother nurtures in her daughter; cf. Olson (2008b: 147–148) on the adornment of young Roman girls.

At *ll.*18–22, the desires of the *tenerae puellae* are catalogued:

(i) Gilded dresses. The women want their bodies swathed in beautiful fabric. The verb, *tegere* ('to swathe' or 'to cover'), does not suggest modesty but the desire for more fabric because it equates to more gold. In terms of the type of gold dresses to which Ovid refers, the process and artistry were impressive, as Cleland et al (2008: 83) discuss: 'Gold might be directly incorporated in Greek and Roman fabric and dress using metallic thread ... or applied as metal decorations ... Such threads could be woven into the cloth or embroidered onto it: remains of cloth from early Etruscan tombs suggest gold was already being sewn on – like sequins – as discs or other designs in the seventh century BC.'

(ii) Scented hair styled in various ways. Part of *cultus* is aroma, so the hair must be adorned not only with what can be seen, and thus what is visually appealing, but also with what is not seen, but which tantalizes with sweet smells (cf. Lilja 1972). The desire to change one's hair, to experiment with different styles, also preoccupies women. More detailed discussions of hair are to be found in the Commentaries on *Am.* 1.14 and *AA* 3.137–168, 235–250 (below).

(iii) Hands admired for their precious stones. Beautiful hands are not enough; as the body must be swathed in gold-trimmed fabric, the hair perfumed and styled, hands must be adorned with gemstones. As Ovid uses a generic term, *gemmae* ('precious stones'), he evokes the many insets available for rings.

According to Ogden (1992: 35): 'The stones used in jewellery … range right across the mineral kingdom … From about the beginning of the Hellenistic period, and probably connected with Alexander the Great's victories in the East, brighter, transparent stones became more favoured.' Ogden notes the popularity of emeralds as well as 'diamonds, sapphires, aquamarines, peridots, citrines and amethysts' (Ibid. 36); cf. also, Spier (1992) (on extensive examples of rings from the early imperial period) and d'Ambrosio (2001) (on Pompeian rings). For ancient sources on gems, cf. Theophrastus *On Stones* and Pliny Book 37.

(iv) Necks adorned with gems from the East. As with the generic term *gemmae* in relation to the stones in rings, a similar all-purpose term is employed here – *lapides* ('gems') – but with the specification that they come from the East. Ovid undoubtedly has in mind pearls, as those imported from the Persian Gulf were fashionable during this period (cf. Higgins 1980: 174–175). On the value and prestige of pearls, cf. Pliny 9.54.

(v) Ears bedecked with gems; cf. *AA* 129–130 (p. 109); also p. 16.

The list is introduced at *l*.18 by *vultis* ('you want'), which indicates that these women have agency; the verb implies a sense of purpose and determination (accentuated by its repetition at *ll*.18–20). Through these emphases on the women's active desires (or demands) for personal luxury items, Ovid employs a motif of Augustan literature, namely that of the past and its contrast to the present. For example, unlike the dutiful Sabine girl, who sees to her flock, tends the fields, obeys her parents and wants for nothing, Ovid's *puellae* are not hard working but, nevertheless, have high expectations.

As Rosati (1985: 66) notes, Ovid's list of female 'must haves' matches the *topoi* of Roman invective against women, expressly in comedy and satire. Even in *AA* 3.129–134 (p. 109), Ovid is somewhat censorious in his advice about female luxury and facets of adornment, but this is mild in comparison to other authors. More biting is *Rem*. 301–302 on the demanding girl who has 'this and that' but is never satisfied because she is greedy – an image suited to the satiric nature of the poem.

At this point in the poem, the impression is that women embellish themselves for the benefit of the gaze of others, implicitly the male gaze (in the expansion of the Ovidian definition of *cultus* and *forma* at *ll*.29–34, it is further argued that women also adorn themselves for their own benefit). At *ll*.23–24,

Ovid reassures his audience that adornments are not *indigna* ('unworthy' 'unbecoming', 'shameful') – women must take care to please the well-groomed men of the era. The word Ovid uses for these fashion-conscious *viri* ('men') is the participle *compti* from the verb *comere* (lit. 'to pay attention to one's hair'; also 'to adorn' and, as translated, 'well-groomed'). Ovid extends the topic of men's interest in adornment in *ll.*25–26 with a vivid flourish; husbands mimic femininity and can even rival a *nupta* ('wife') in terms of *cultus*. Ovid's use of *mariti* ('husbands') reveals something of the specificities of his audience; he composes, in part, for married women, that is, respectable women. Thus, in his view, refinement is as much a part of a married woman's world as it is of the unmarried. The imagery of marriage and married life, evoked by references to the *maritus* ('husband') and *nupta*, combined with acknowledgement of men's interest in *cultus*, indicates that there are married couples who are equal in terms of their immaculate appearance and love of *cultus*.

Ovid employs the adjective *feminea* ('womanly') at *l.*25, which is traditionally a negative description of a man. To compare a male's appearance with that of a woman is usually accompanied by ridicule, particularly accusations of *mollitia*; cf., for some examples, Cicero *Against Verres* 2.5.31 and *Against Catiline* 2.22–23; Seneca the Younger *Epistle* 122.7–8; Martial 1.96 and 3.74; Quintilian *Institutes of Oratory* 5.9.14. The reasons for Ovid's position here are twofold:

(i) Rhetorical strategy. Ovid's primary goal is to instruct women in the art of beautification by persuading them to try a recipe or two. Therefore, an effective tactic is to draw attention to their cultivated husbands by employing exaggeration.

(ii) The Ovidian persona. The poetic voice of the *Medicamina* belongs to a man from a sophisticated social milieu, seemingly unconcerned with paying deference to rigid gender binaries. Such a man, indicative of a new breed of men in the late-first century BC, is evoked in the words of Vout (1996: 212):

> [V]ictorious Romans could not live in less luxury than the nations they had conquered. We can scarcely imagine that they would have been content to wear a heavy, white toga which had changed little over the centuries, when there were embroidered silks on offer.

This argument is supplemented by her inclusion of the perceptive words of Lurie: 'The wearing of a single foreign garment, like the dropping of a foreign word or phrase in conversation is meant ... to indicate sophistication. It can also mean advertising wealth.' (Lurie 1981: 12–13).

## Lines 27–28 – corrupt lines

The problems of the lines and the attempts to repair them are addressed on p. 137. In keeping with Kenney's assessment, the lines remain obelized; yet it should be noted that part of *l.*27, after appropriate punctuation following *refert*, leaves the perfectly workable – *Munditia crimina nulla meret* – 'Simple elegance warrants no reproaches.' This does not help, however, with the rest of the couplet, which has been subject to some ingenious, if strained efforts to make it work, none of which are compelling.

## Lines 29–34 – *cultus* and *forma*

Ovid provides three examples to expand upon the themes of *cultus* and *forma*:

(i) Even country women style their *comae* ('tresses'). Ovid subverts the stereotype of country folk as simple, rough and unsophisticated – cultivated women (*cultae*) can even be found in the wilderness. The imagery of wild countryside is evoked by the reference to Athos, a mountain on the easternmost of the promontories of Chalcidice in the northern Aegean. It represents remoteness, ruggedness (because of its thick forest) and loftiness (reaching a height of 2033 metres). He employs the image elsewhere; cf., for example, *Met.* 2.216–217 and *Ep.* 1.5.22.

(ii) Love of oneself, care of oneself, is a source of delight (*voluptas*), and beauty (*forma*) certainly delights young girls. An evocative word in the Latin erotic vocabulary, *voluptas* is regularly associated with sexual activities or sexuality per se; Ovid uses it at *Am.*1.10.35 and *Met.* 4.327. Adams (1982: 197–198) associates it with *gaudium* ('delight'). Again Ovid subverts the norm – one can experience *voluptas* by pleasing oneself – beautification (or *cultus*) is for the delight of the individual here, not for the pleasure of another's gaze.

(iii) Juno's bird, the peacock. The peacock wears star-like spots on its tail, the eyes of Argus, placed by Hera after the giant was slain by Hermes; cf. *Met.*

1.722–723 and 15.385. The peacock epitomizes the poet's views on *forma* and *voluptas*: beauty can give pleasure to others (as the peacock's unfurled tail brings to mankind) *and* to oneself (the peacock exults in its own magnificence). The choice of verb here, *superbire*, literally means 'to be haughty' as well as 'to take pride' (here translated as 'exults'). It is a powerful word, regularly with negative connotations, used here to champion *cultus* and its connection to justifiable self-exaltation. On the idea of beauty breeding arrogance, cf. *Am.* 2.17 on Corinna's beauty.

## Lines 35–42 – Witchcraft

The previous three examples (*ll*.29–34) lead to another Ovidian maxim: men are inspired by *amor* – not magic. This in turn introduces a new topic: witchcraft. Like other Augustan poets, Ovid often refers to magic and witches; cf. Tibullus 1.5 and 2.6; Propertius 1.1; Horace *Satire* 1.8 and *Epodes* 5 and 17. He has a poem on the witch / *lena*, Dipsas (*Am.* 1.8) and makes various references to magic throughout his works (cf., for example, *Her.* 12; *Ars* 2.99ff.; *Rem.* 249–290; *Met.* Books 7 and 14). Belief in the efficacy of magic for securing the man or woman of your dreams was widespread throughout the ancient world, leaving behind a substantial archaeological and written record. Ovid does not believe in such practices but the passage nevertheless demonstrates his knowledge of the topic. That magic is something to avoid is stressed by the repetition of *nec* ('not') at *ll*.37–40, each time occupying emphatic placement as the first word of the line.

At *ll*.35–36 erotic magic is introduced via the reference to *fortes herbae* ('powerful herbs'). Herbal ingredients were commonplace in magic and their effectiveness was believed to be enhanced if they were procured according to specific instructions; for example, being gathered on a certain calendar day and / or at a particular time. In view of the recipes that follow, the lines on magic may not be an unnecessary poetic flourish but rather a means by which the poet can establish legitimacy for his *medicamina*. Far from magical nonsense with silly and dangerous ingredients, his recipes for feminine beauty, and thus desirability, are sensible, effective and non-lethal. Indicative of the symbiosis between medicine, science, cosmeceuticals and magic in antiquity, Ovid's recipes are to be regarded as discrete from witches' brews.

Several magical practices are mentioned:

(i) Mixtures of grasses and juices of unspecified ingredients. *gramina* ('grasses', 'herbs' or 'leaves'); *suci* ('juices', 'saps' and also 'potions').

(ii) A baneful potion. The word for potion is *virus*, which has connotations of something slimy, foul of taste and malodorous; thus, it also designates poison. This particular potion, according to Ovid, is composed of a substance from a mare on heat, which is a reference to the *hippomanes*, a famous aphrodisiac in antiquity. Aristotle defines the substance as a black, viscous compound on the forehead of a newborn foal and also as a secretion from a mare (*History of Animals* 572a–b, 577a). He notes that both types of *hippomanes* were sought by those manufacturing spells. Theocritus references it as a plant that sends horses mad (*Idyll* 2.48–49) and Dioscorides (2.173) also identifies it as a plant (the caper). Clearly Ovid's expression, *amans equa* ('a mare on heat') indicates he understood *hippomanes* to be a mare's sexual secretion (as does Virgil in *Georgics* 3.280–283), while at *AA* 2.100, Ovid takes *hippomanes* to be the substance from the foal's forehead. Cf. Tupet (1986: 2653–2656); Watson (1993) and above (p. 56).

(iii) Splitting snakes with Marsian spells. Ovid tells us (*AA* 2.102) that the Marsi, a formidable tribe from central Italy to the south-east of Rome, were renowned for incantations and magic; he places them in the same company as Medea and Circe. The Marsi were also snake-handlers or snake-charmers. Silius Italicus (*Punica* 8.495–497) writes of the Marsi chanting to snakes, causing them to fall asleep, while Lucilius (*Fragment* 605–606 Warmington) claims the chanting caused the snakes to explode. Further on exploding snakes, cf. Lucian *The Lover of Lies* ll.11–13 and, on the Marsi and this skill, Pliny 28.28. Cf. Horace *Epode* 17.29 where Canidia has induced a headache that afflicts him, which is described as a form of Marsian magic.

(iv) Sorceresses reversing water flow. In both Greek and Roman belief, witches were thought to have the power to interfere in the natural world; cf. *Met.* 7.198–202. In his arresting passage on Thessalian witches, Lucan (*Civil War* 6.461–484) lists examples of their interferences in nature, including altering water courses.

(v) Temese in southern Italy had copper mines from which metal cymbals were manufactured – hence Ovid's Temesaean bronze. The clanging of cymbals was a form of apotropaic magic to counter witches' attempts to draw down the moon (cf. *Met.* 7.207–209). The metaphor is a sly, somewhat obtuse one: people can set aside their cymbals without fear as the efforts of apotropaic magic are redundant because witches *cannot* draw down the moon. In other words: magic is hokum.

Ovid refers to the moon as Luna, an ancient Italic divinity, rather than her Greco-Roman embodiment, Artemis / Diana, while the image of the goddess in her chariot is standard in poetry. The premise behind drawing down the moon was associated most commonly with erotic magic; motivated by the witch's desire to collect the juice that dripped from the lowered moon (cf. Apuleius *Metamorphoses* 1.3). On witches drawing down the moon, cf. Horace *Epode* 5.45–46 and Lucan 6.499–506; for Greek sources, cf. Aristophanes *Clouds* 746–757 and Plato *Gorgias* 513a. Cf. also Watson and Watson (219): 'the banging of various implements … was thought to drive off malignant influences associated with the eclipse … of the moon.' On the latter, cf. also Tupet (1976: 39–43); Hill (1973). On magic in antiquity, including erotic magic, cf. Winkler (1991); Faraone (1999); Edmonds (2013).

## Lines 43–50 – Beauty fades

Ovid advises the *puellae* about inner beauty and the need to nurture one's character as well as one's face. At *l.*43 he instructs them to be conscious of their moral fibre (*mos*) and at *l.*44 to be mindful of their character (*ingenium*). One cares for oneself, shows respect for oneself, by cultivating the outside as well as the inside, and presenting an image to the world that is as good as it can possibly be. In this sense, *cultus* extends to integrity and grace – good looks and an appealing character make an irresistible combination.

The theme of ageing and its physical effects introduced in *l.*45 is accentuated by the imagery at *l.*46: features (*vultus*) that were once pleasing will be ploughed (*arare*) by wrinkles (*rugae*, also at *l.*48). Warming to his theme, in order to stress the need for inner-cultivation and perhaps as a selling point for the recipes that follow, Ovid notes the emotional pain accompanying an ageing exterior. Gazing at oneself in a *speculum* ('mirror') will be a source of displeasure and the resultant *dolor* ('grief') at one's ageing reflection will cause even more wrinkles.

On the sorrows of ageing, Ovid follows a long line of Greek and Roman poets. The Homeric epics include epithets such as *stugeron* ('hateful'; *Iliad* 19.336) and *khalepon* ('harsh'; *Iliad* 8.103, 23.623; *Odyssey* 11.196) for old age (cf. Bertman 1989: 159). In the *Homeric Hymn to Aphrodite* (*ll.*218–238), the goddess tells the story of Eos and Tithonos, unquestionably the most powerful myth pertaining to the hideousness and hopelessness of ageing in the Greco-Roman world. In *Poem* 58, for example, Sappho contemplates the myth as she considers the beauty of youth in contrast to her own old age. Mimnermus, composing earlier, produced some of the most intense lamentations on the isolation, despair and humiliation that accompanies the onset of old age. Such themes, with an emphasis on old women, are treated by later poets and scattered throughout the *Greek Anthology* (for a few examples: 5.21, 5.28, 5.76, 5.103, 5.112, 5.204, 11.67 and 11.69). In the latter sources and the more infamous Latin poems on the same topic (cf. Horace *Epodes* 8 and 12), old age incites intense anxiety and, regularly, repulsion. On ageing in Greek and Roman literature and society, cf. Falkner and de Luce (1989); Falkner (1996); Cokayne (2003); Parkin (2003).

The proem concludes with a final piece of advice (*ll.*49–50), which essentially constitutes a repetition of the subject matter of the previous six lines. At *l.*49 Ovid uses one of the strongest value terms in the Latin vocabulary, *probitas* ('probity', 'moral uprightness', 'rectitude'). According to Ovid, *probitas* endures and ultimately nurtures *amor*. A frequent word in Ovid's exile poetry, *probitas* is used especially in connection with his own wife and is a term applied to the exemplary wife per se (though it is also used of men). Johnson (1997: 412) observes that *probitas* appears only twice in the pre-exile works 'where it is diametrically opposed to beauty'; one is the passage from the *Med.* and the other is Helen's words to Paris in the *Heroides* (17.173–174):

> De facie metuit, vitae confidit, et illum
>   securum probitas, forma timere facit.

> As for my face [*facies*] it frightens him, he is trusting of my ways, and
>   my probity [*probitas*] makes him secure, my beauty [*forma*] scares him.

In the exile poems, *probitas* appears in relation to Ovid's wife:

*Epistle* 3.1.93–94:

Nota tua est probitas testataque tempus in omne;
   sit virtus etiam non probitate minor.

Your probity [*probitas*] is known and proven for all time;
   let your virtue [*virtus*] be no less than your probity [*probitas*].

*Tristia* 5.14.21–28:

Nam tua, dum stetimus, turpi sine crimine mansit,
   et tantum probitas inreprehensa fuit.
Area de nostra nunc est tibi facta ruina;
   conspicuum virtus hic tua ponat opus.
Esse bonam facile est, ubi quod vetet esse remotum est,
   et nihil officio nupta quod obstet habet.
Cum deus intonuit non se subducere nimbo,
   id demum est pietas, id socialis amor.

For your true probity [*probitas*], while I stood strong,
   remained free from ugly accusation and was above reproach.
Now a space has been created for you on account of our ruin;
   here let your virtue [*virtus*] set down a visible structure.
It is easy to be good, when what forbids it is remote,
   and a wife [*nupta*] has nothing to get in the way of her duties.
Not to avoid the storm when a god thunders,
   that alone is true piety [*pietas*], that is marital love [*socialis amor*].

## Lines 51–52 – The recipes, an introduction

The first recipe is introduced with a repetition of the opening couplet: the imperative *discite* ('learn') of *l*.1 reappears at *l*.51 as does the promise of beauty. The advice that introduces the first recipe concerns the right time to apply it: after sleep has released *teneri artus* ('tender limbs'), the application will ensure that the face of the *puella* will shine radiantly (*candida*). The modern tone of the couplet is noted by Green (1979: 282): 'His first recipe ... is for a face pack guaranteed to produce a brighter complexion – much like modern advertising for products guaranteed to give women a brighter, fresher complexion.'

Both *tenera* and *candida* are words used of the elegiac *puella*; for Ovid's employment of the terms, cf., for example: Corinna (unnamed) in *Am.* 3.3.25 is *tenera*; in *Her.* 15.216, Cupid has hands described as *teneri* and at *AA* 1.7, Amor is, overall, *tener*; Ovid's verse in *AA* 2.273 is *tener* (cf., also *Am.* 3.8.2); Corinna at *Am.* 1.5.10 has a neck that is *candida* ('radiant'; a reference to Catullus 68.70, in which Lesbia is described as *candida diva* – 'radiant goddess'); Corinna is *candida* at *Am.* 3.3.5; Lampetia likewise shines at *Met.* 2.349, as does Penelope at *Am.* 2.18.29.

## Lines 53–68 – Recipe 1

*Ingredients:*
23 oz (654 g) of Libyan barley with husks and coverings removed
23 oz (654 g) of bitter vetch
10 eggs
2 oz (55 g) of hartshorn
12 narcissus bulbs with the rind removed
2 oz (55 g) of gum
2 oz (55 g) of Tuscan seed
17 oz (491 g) of honey

*Method:*
Step i: Soak the vetch in the eggs
Step ii: Add the barley
Step iii: Dry the ingredients in gusty breezes
Step iv: Have a slow she-ass crush the dry ingredients on a millstone
Step v: Add the narcissus bulbs and hartshorn
Step vi: Sift the mixture
Step vii: Pound the narcissus bulbs on clean marble and add
Step viii: Add the gum and Tuscan seed
Step ix: Add honey

(i) Barley (*hordeum*); cf. also *l*.95; Fig. 7. Green (1979: 383) notes that modern creams do not include barley, but some contain oatmeal or oat-flour that comes from the same family (*Poaceae*). Oat-flour has long been used to treat skin disorders and improve the complexion and the softness of the skin. The anti-inflammatory and anti-pruritic effects of oat components were recognized in antiquity, and oat-based lotions are still used to treat sores and other inflammatory skin conditions as well as various causes of pruritus, including burns, bites and sunburn. Certain phenols in oats also protect the skin from free radical damage and oat-based products have been found to facilitate skin hydration. For a discussion of modern uses and scientific data, cf. Makdisi, Kutner and Friedman (2014).

In Rome barley was incorporated into a variety of remedies, both medicinal and cosmetic, and was prescribed for topical application as well as ingestion. Pliny cites numerous recipes including barley, especially *polenta* (pearl-barley, that is, barley with its hull and bran removed); cf., for example, his face-pack at 20.20:

> Silvestre rapum in arvis maxime nascitur: fruticosum, semine candido, duplo maiore quam papaver. Hoc ad levigandam cutem in facie totoque corpore utuntur mixta farina pari mensura ervi, hordei et tritici et lupini, radix ad omnia inutilis.

> The wild turnip grows best in arable fields: bushy, with a white seed, twice the size of the poppy. Used to smooth the skin on the face or the entire body it is mixed with equal parts of the meal of bitter vetch, barley and wheat and lupins, the root being useless for anything.

Cf. also, Pliny 20.26 (the pounded stalks of white lettuce mixed with pearl-barley and applied with cold water to soothe cramps and sprains; the stalks, when mixed with pearl-barley and wine, assist with the alleviation of pimples); 20.81 (a liniment made with pounded cabbage and other ingredients, including barley flour to medicate gout); 21.129 (narcissus root, honey and pearl-barley mixed with oil to heal bruises and wounds). Celsus lists various uses of barley; cf. for example, pearl-barley as an enema (2.12) and as a poultice for drawing out infections (2.33). Cf. also Winter (2009: 98) on the continuation of the use of pearl-barley, particularly by Chinese herbalists. The ingredient is used again in the fifth recipe (*l*.95).

(ii) Bitter vetch (*ervum*) is a species of the genus *Vicia*; cf. Fig. 8. A member of the legume family (*Fabaceae*), vetch is one of the oldest crops in the ancient

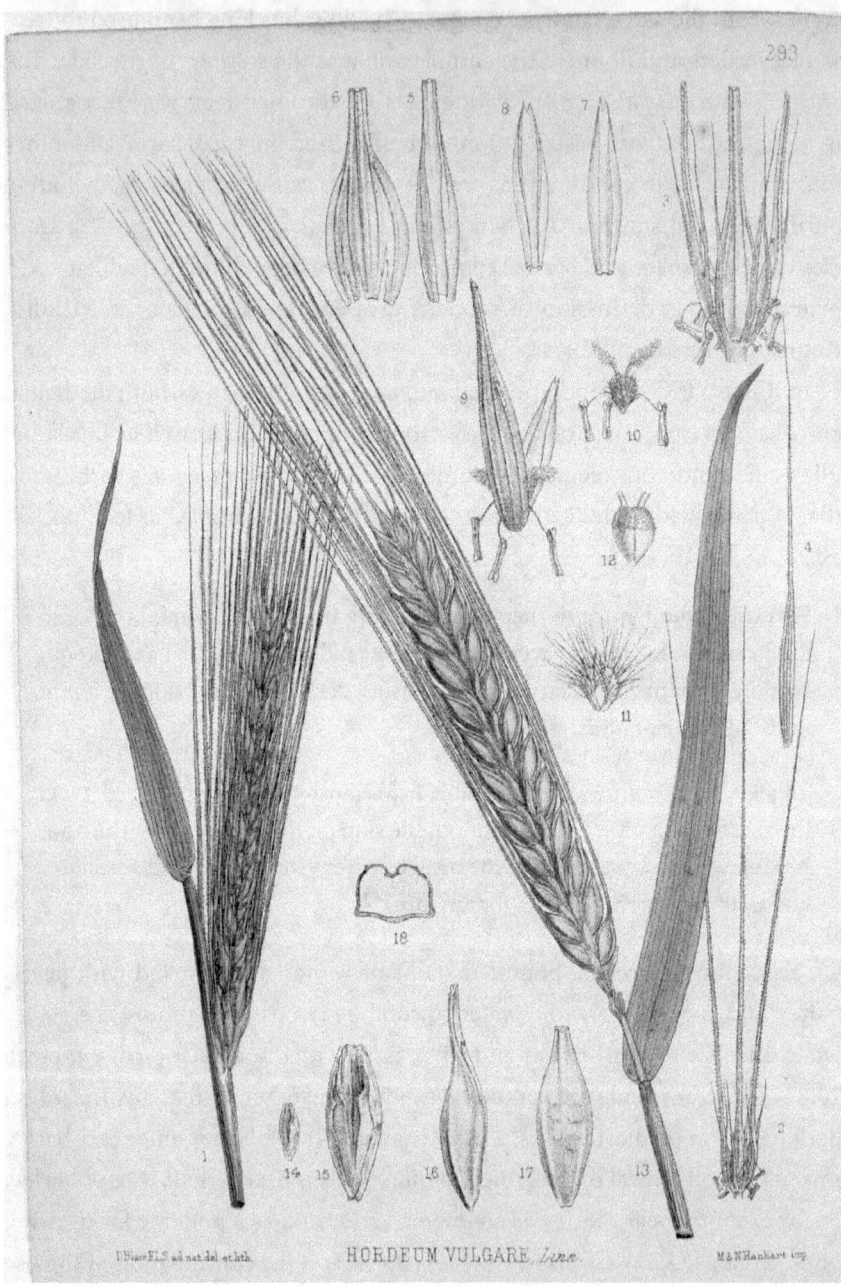

**Fig. 7** Barley (*Hordeum vulgare*).

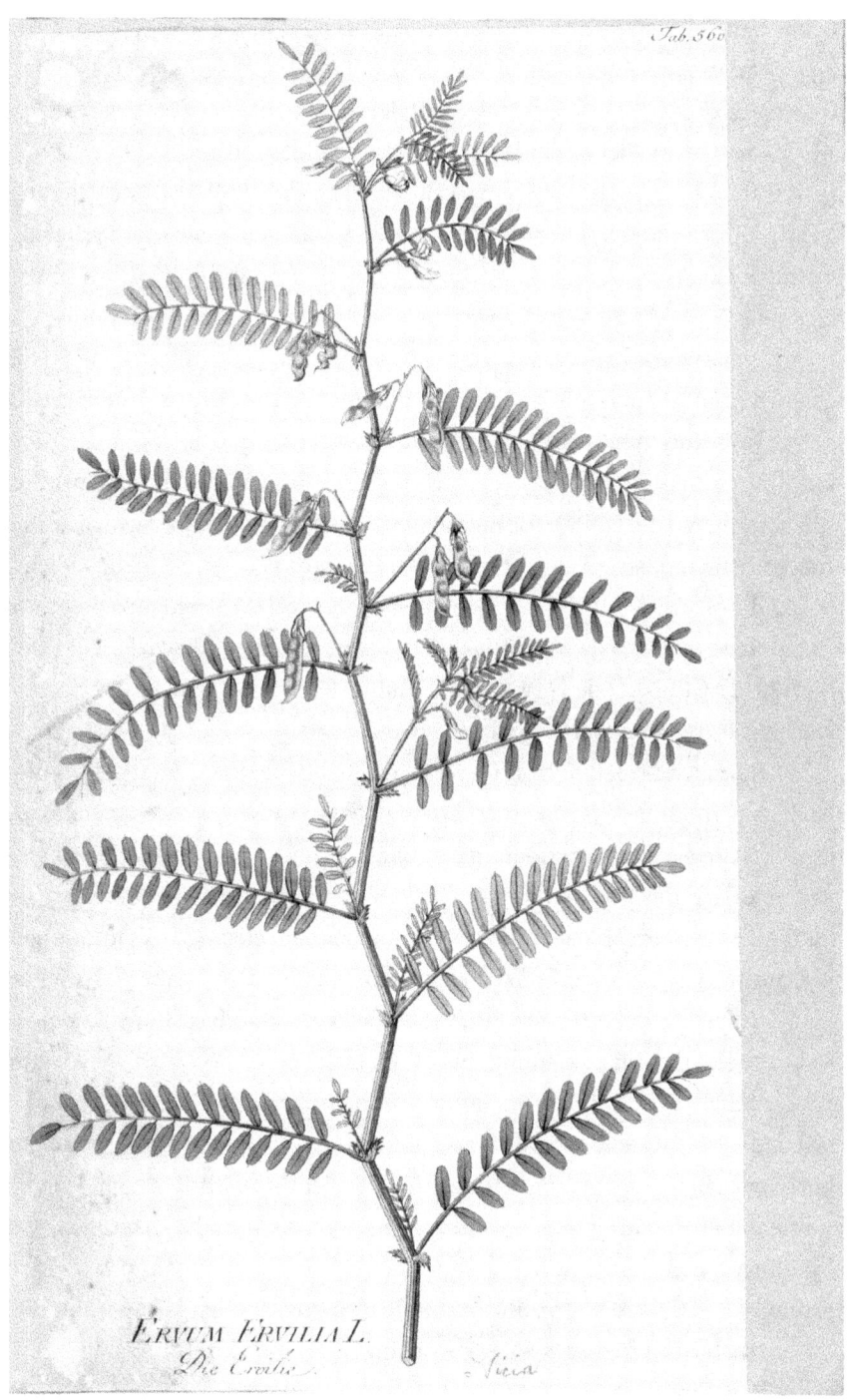

**Fig. 8** Bitter vetch (*Ervum ervilia* [sic]).

Mediterranean; its seeds resemble red lentils and, as its name suggests, it is unpleasant to taste. According to Winter (2009: 386), the ingredient was added to cosmetic creams as a thickening agent; it is also an effective emollient. Pliny cites its use in medicinal and beautification recipes; on the latter, cf. 20.20 (p. 61); cf. also 22.151 for its remarkably widespread applications (including healing bites, removing pimples, blemishes, boils and chilblains, and relieving pruritus). Cf. also Celsus 2.33 on bitter vetch in a poultice for drawing out infections; 5.5 and 5.16 as a cleanser.

(iii) Egg (*ovum*) is a common, all-purpose ingredient in antiquity and is still included in modern, home-made facial treatments. The purpose and benefits of eggs in beauty treatments are well known, for example: for tightening the skin, thus softening wrinkles (egg white); for stimulating circulation, thus enhancing glow (egg white); adding moisture (yolk). In modern pharmaceutical and cosmetic industries, eggs are widely used; in relation to cosmetic creams, the lipid (oils, fats and waxes) content of the yolk is recognized for its moisturizing quality as well as its emulsifying properties; cf. Laca, Paredes and Díaz (2012). Cf. also Galen (14.422–423 Kühn 1827) who has a facial recipe for cleansing and toning that includes egg white.

(iv) Hartshorn (*cornu cervinum*) was originally obtained by distilling the shavings of the antlers (sometimes also the hoofs) of a stag. When crystallized, the substance becomes ammonium carbonate, an ammonium salt, and an early version of baking powder. Today, the powder is industrially produced by heating ammonium chloride (Ovid's Ammoniac salt; cf. p. 78) or ammonium sulphate with calcium carbonate. Hartshorn was used in healing as well as beautification products. Green (1979: 384) suggests that hartshorn was most likely burned, the ash containing 'quicklime (calcium oxide), with phosphates and carbonates, including ammonium carbonate'; cf. Pliny 28.178 (pp. 117–118) and 28.187. Calcium oxide is still used today in products that cleanse the skin (lifting dirt from pores and stimulating circulation for a bright complexion) and treat hair (for straightening and waving, and also in some shampoos). Cf. also Pliny 28.233 on the use of hartshorn in the relief of pruritus and 28.241 for cleaning sores; Celsus 3.20 on burning hartshorn to cure lethargy and insomnia.

Note that the ingredients are to be the first antlers to fall from a stag. These instructions show the connection between cosmeceuticals, some medical traditions and, most likely, magic in the form of homeopathy. As the recipe is for improving the skin, the specification of the first antlers suggests the concept of *similia similibus curantur* ('like cures like'); namely, to achieve a youthful complexion, ingredients need to be 'youthful'. On homeopathy in antiquity, particularly in medicine, cf. Shapiro and Shapiro (1997).

(v) Narcissus bulb (*narcissi bulbus*); cf. Fig. 9. The preparation of the narcissus bulb for lotions, particularly ones targeting pimples, sores and other causes of skin discomfort, has a long history throughout antiquity, continuing to the present day. Celsus (5.6) includes the bulb in an extensive list of erodents (including myrrh, frankincense and uncooked honey) and also lists it as an emollient (5.15). Pliny (21.129) discusses the use of narcissus: when mixed with honey, it helps to heal wounds and burns; the latter mix, combined with darnel, medicates superficial abscesses. Dioscorides (4.158) lists several uses: with honey it heals burns, sores around tendons, ankle sprains and joint pain; mixed with nettle seed and vinegar, it removes freckles and white leprosies. Some modern body lotions include the liquid extract from the bulb of *Narcissus tazetta* to assist in preserving moisture content.

To obtain the narcissus gum, Ovid specifies that it must be pounded on marble that is 'pure' in respect of its state of cleanliness; cf. Horace *Epistle* 1.2.54 where he states that a jar must be clean otherwise the contents become sour. Leary (1988a: 25) and Saiko (2005: 205–206) suggest that the marble is most likely a mortar and pestle. Saiko further suggests that the purity to which Ovid refers may indicate a general sense of cleanliness – not only in regard to equipment – but also ingredients; that is, everything needs to be cleaned so that impurities do not get into the preparation process.

(vi) Gum (*gummi* = *cummi*). Ovid omits details as to what type of gum to use, although it may have been gum arabic (cf. Saiko 2005: 206), imported from the Near East and North Africa, or gum tragacanth from the shrub goatsthorn in Greece and Asia Minor (cf. Dirckx 1980: 330). Green (1979: 389) suggests that gum may have given the mixture an astringent quality and cites Pliny 24.106 (who writes that gums improve complexion). Gum arabic is used as an emulsifier and dispersing agent in modern products, including moisturizers, shampoos, wash gels, soaps and mascara.

(vii) Tuscan seed (*semen Tuscum*). Most likely *Triticum spelta*, a variety of common wheat, native to the Mediterranean, including Etruria, and one of the oldest domesticated cereal. Related to wheat (*Triticum aestivum*), from which

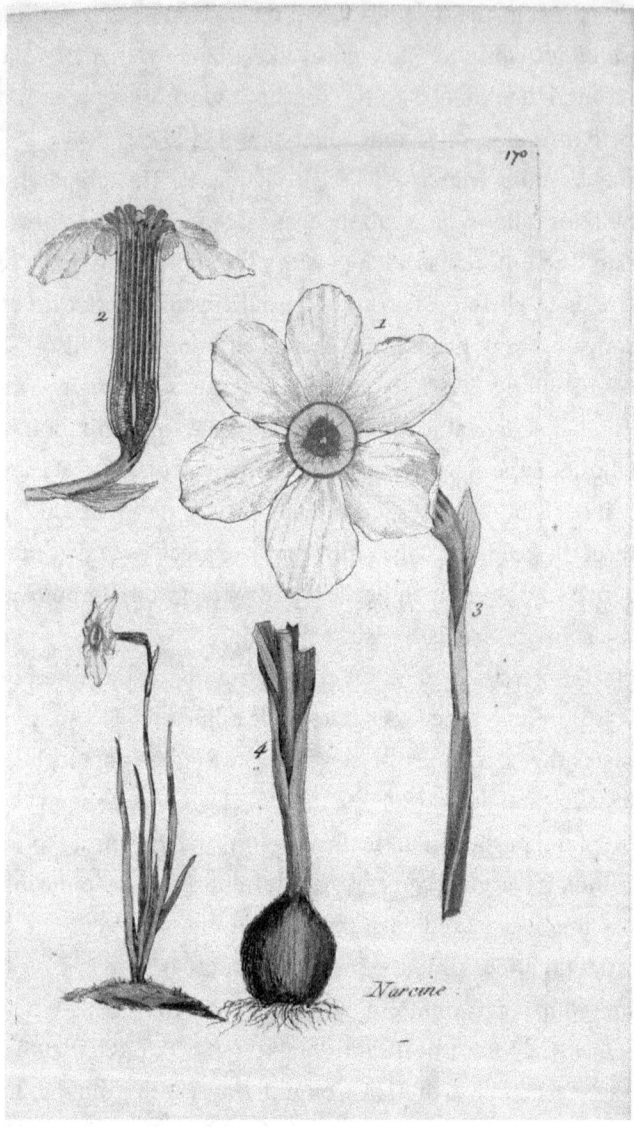

**Fig. 9** Narcissus (*Flora Parisiensis*).

is extracted wheat germ oil (containing lecithin and fatty acids), known to have emollient properties and for this reason used in cosmetics, the oil of *Triticum spelta* is used in various body lotions, facial creams and bath products; cf. above p. 61 for Pliny's inclusion of *Triticum* in a face-pack.

(viii) Honey (*mel*). An age-old beauty product, particularly as an emulsifier, honey is used in numerous recipes for both healing and beautification. Attic honey was regarded as the best, with that from Mt Hymettus being especially prized as its taste was enhanced by the thyme on which the bees fed. Honey is also an antibacterial: Theophrastus in *Enquiry into Plants* observes that mixtures including honey are effective in the healing of wounds and also sores on the head (9.9), tumours (9.11) and burns (9.19). Celsus (5.16) recommends honey as a skin cleanser, suggesting that if mixed with an ingredient such as bitter vetch it is more effective. Cf. Pliny 16.71 on a mixture including honey for the treatment of sore eyes; 18.61 on wild poppy and honey for throat diseases; 20.4 with wild cucumber for extreme tonsillitis causing abscesses on the throat. For beautification of the skin, cf. Pliny 20.23 on a mixture of garlic and honey to improve the ill-effects of liver-spots; 30.10 on a mixture of lanolin and Corsican honey to remove spots on the face and also a mixture of rose oil and honey on wool to remove dead skin cells on the face (that is, as an exfoliate for a brighter complexion). Saiko (2005: 206) mentions the practicality of including honey because of its spreadability. Cf. Cilliers and Retief (2008); Burlando and Cornara (2013); Majno (1975: 117–118).

At *ll.*67–68, Ovid promises that this *medicamen* ('treatment') will result in a *vultus* ('face') that will gleam more smoothly than a mirror, implying a symbiosis between woman and mirror. Additionally, the mirror, a key object in a woman's toilette, is, like the finished product of the adornment it assists, an object of beauty. The woman will eventually put down the mirror and end her self-reflexive gaze and, upon leaving her boudoir, will 'see' herself in the 'mirror' of others as they respond to her gleaming face. On the mirror in the *Med.*, cf. Rimell (2006: 178 and 194); cf. also Figs 3 and 4.

## Lines 69–76 – Recipe 2

*Ingredients:*
69 oz (1962 g) roasted lupin-seeds
69 oz (1962 g) fried beans
0.3 oz (9 g) white lead
0.3 oz (9 g) red natron scum
0.3 oz (9 g) iris from Illyrica

*Method:*
Step i: Roast the lupin-seeds
Step ii: Fry the beans
Step iii: Refine the ingredients on a rough millstone
Step iv: Combine, in equal amounts, white lead, red natron scum and iris
Step v: Give the above ingredients to strong-armed young men to be pounded
Step vi: Combine the ground lupins, ground beans and 1 oz (27 g) of the pounded mixture

(i) Lupin-seeds (*lupinus*); cf. Fig. 10. The lupin is a legume of the *Fabaceae* family. It is likely that Ovid meant for the seeds to be used as they were a common commodity derived from the plant. Dioscorides (2.109) recommends lupin meal as a skin cleanser and medicant for spots; when boiled with rain water, the thickened paste cleanses the face. Celsus (5.28) lists lupin meal as an ingredient to medicate scabies and Pliny provides various medical poultices and cleansers that include lupins (22.154–157; 32.87). Lupin oil, extracted from the seeds, is contained in some modern moisturizers and is promoted by some companies as possessing anti-ageing properties because it stimulates the production of collagen.

That the lupin-seeds must be pale may be an example of signatures (a plant or other ingredient has characteristics of its intended application). In this context, as Rimell (2006: 198) has noted: 'Qualities belonging to ingredients are to be transferred to the female face: thus lupin seeds . . . are pale, like the girl's desired complexion, just like the white lead combined with the blush of red nitre in line 73.'

(ii) Beans (*fabae*). Ovid uses *faba*, possibly the broad bean, which is in fact from the pea family. The *faba* was a popular ingredient in the Roman diet, with an entire section dedicated to it in Apicius's *The Art of Cooking* (5.4). The broad bean is still used in facial and body creams because of its high quality, nourishing oil. The beans may have been included to make the skin look 'plump' and thereby healthy.

(iii) White lead (*cerussa*). When one thinks about ancient cosmetics, lead is something that often comes to mind. White lead was used by painters as well as cosmeticians; it was also medicinal and, when ingested or applied topically in large quantities, poisonous. The dangers of lead were known to Pliny (34.167;

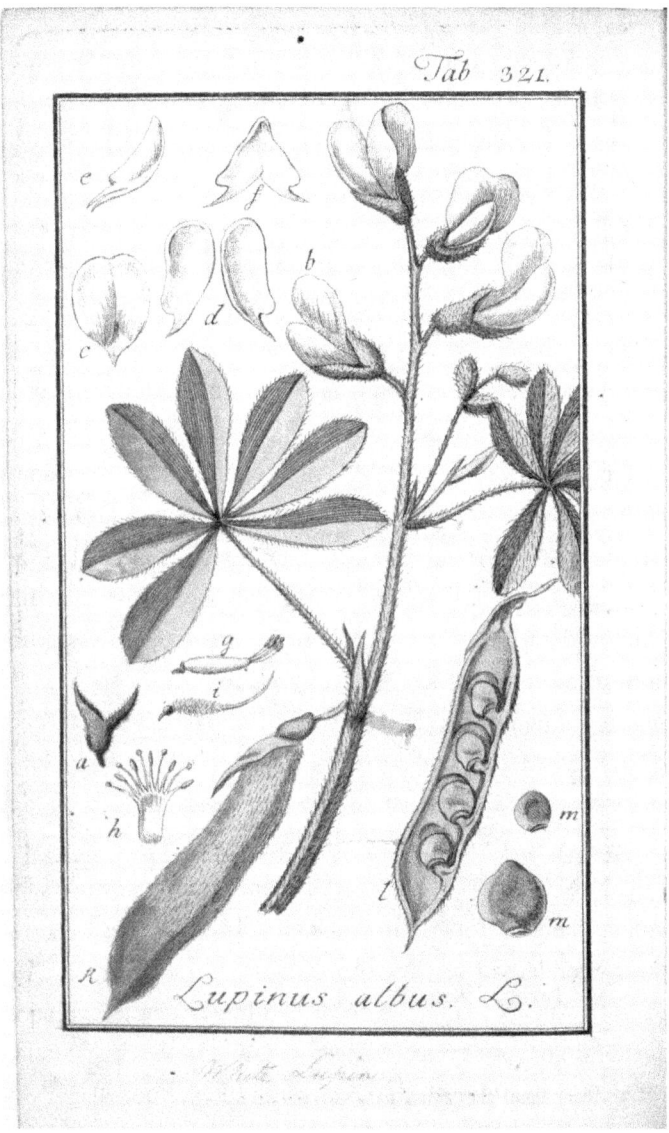

**Fig. 10** White lupin (*Lupinus albus*).

34.175), Vitruvius (*On Architecture* 8.6) and Dioscorides (5.88). For cosmeceutical and cosmetic purposes, white lead was manufactured in antiquity by pouring vinegar over lead shavings to dissolve them. The mixture was dried, ground and made into small cakes that were sold commercially (Olson 2009: 295). It was usually applied as a foundation after cleansing and moisturizing, although in this recipe it is used as an emulsifier; cf. Martial 1.72, 2.41.11–12 and 7.25 on references to white lead as a foundation. Cf. Shear (1936), who discusses cosmetic jars containing traces of *psimythion* (lead carbonate), which had been deposited in the graves of Greek women and girls of the fifth and fourth centuries BC.

(iv) Ruddy natron scum (*nitri spuma rubentis*). Natron is a mineral predominately comprised of sodium carbonate decahydrate (hydrated soda ash or soda crystals) that occurs naturally in saline river beds. While its colour is white, it may be described here as ruddy because of the discolouring effects of iron bacteria in the water. In Egypt, natron was harvested from dry lake beds and used in a variety of products from medicines, insecticides and as a drying agent in the mummification process. As it softens water while removing dirt and grease, hydrated soda scum makes an effective skin cleanser.

(v) Illyrian iris (*Iris illyrica*). Ovid does not mention the part of the plant to be used, although it is almost certainly orris root. Dioscorides specifies that the root is employed regularly; cf. 1.1 where he provides a description of the preparation of the roots, which are cut, dried in a shady spot and stored by being hung from linen thread. He also specifies that the best plants come from Illyria as well as Macedonia, listing a variety of medicinal applications, including a mixture of iris and white hellebore to minimise freckles and heal sunburn. Celsus (5.15) recommends iris and honey for a skin cleanser and Pliny (21.143) discusses uses for the red iris, both as an ingestible substance, as well as an ingredient for topical mixtures for sores, abscesses, corns and warts. If the bulb is intended for use here, it would provide a cleansing effect, which, combined with the roasted lupin-seeds (adding a gentle exfoliant), would ensure a thorough yet gentle cleanser overall. If the iris petals are also incorporated, they would scent the cream with the perfume usually defined as the scent of 'sweet violet' or 'essence of violet' (cf. Green 1979: 386n45).

At *l*.75, the recipe specifies that the white lead, ruddy natron scum and iris are to be pounded (*subigere*) by the strong (*validi*) arms of young men (*iuvenes*), recalling *l*.64 and the instructions to grind (*terere*) the narcissus bulbs with a 'vigorous right-hand'. Watson (2001: 459) rightly observes that the youths mentioned are slaves. *subigere* has agricultural connotations of ploughing or cultivating, as well as kneading. As Adams (1982: 155) notes, the verb is also implicitly sexual, designating 'the active role in homosexual or heterosexual intercourse, in which sense it was probably established in ordinary speech'. Adams (Ibid.) cites the use of the verb in a bawdy military song quoted by Suetonius (*Caesar* 49.4); for further discussion, cf. Adams (1982: 155–156). *terere*, translated at *l*.64 as 'grind', also has an agricultural meaning, such as rubbing grain from ears by thrashing or treading. According to Adams (Ibid. 183), in certain contexts, *terere* has various sexual implications related to acts of rubbing and stimulating, including masturbation. However, in the line of the *Med.*, while there is clearly an overtly sexual implication due to the imagery of the young men with their muscular arms pounding away, the word *terere* also means to cleanse or beautify by pounding something till it is smooth or shiny. Ovid's brawny youths are envisaged as assisting in the woman's beautification process by pounding her (ingredients).

As recipes one and two produce substantial quantities, the mixtures would have been stored in either one large container and portioned into smaller vessels as required, or distributed into several small containers. In Fig. 1 an example of a personal canister is represented. Measuring 6 cm in diameter and 5.2 cm in height and dated to the mid-second century AD, the canister was discovered in an archaeological site in London. Scientific tests conducted on the contents concluded that the substance was made from animal fat and the starch of plant roots or grains. The white cream was described as 'slightly granular' with a 'pleasant texture when rubbed into the skin' (Evershed et al 2004: 35). Scientists also recorded that while the cream felt 'greasy' on initial contact, 'this was quickly overtaken by the smooth, powdery texture created by the starch.' (Ibid.).

## Lines 77–82 – Recipe 3

*Ingredients:*
0.5 oz (14 g) of *alcyonea*
Attic honey

*Method:*
Step i: Mix the ingredients
Step ii: Apply to the face (if there are spots) and / or to the body

At *ll*.77–78, Ovid refers to *medicamina* ('treatments') sourced from the nest of birds, which are called *alcyonea*. Combined with Attic honey, the paste removes spots; cf. Galen (12.421 Kühn 1826) for a recipe including heated *alcyonea*, honey and a cereal paste for cleansing (also 14.536 Kühn 1827).

The exact nature of *alcyonea* has, at times, proved to be a scholarly conundrum, which has not been assisted by the accounts of ancient authors. Aristotle (*History of Animals* 616a) provides a vague description, associating it generally with all that comprises the light red nest of kingfishers. Hippocrates (*Diseases of Women* 1.106) recommends it be combined with wine for an effective depilation lotion that leaves the skin with a red tinge and looking healthy, but he does not define the substance. Pliny (32.86–87) lists four categories:

> Fit in mari alcyoneum appellatum, e nidis, ut aliqui existumant, alcyonum et ceycum, ut alii, sordibus spumarum crassescentibus, alii e limo vel quadam maris languine. Quattuor eius genera: cinereum, spissum, odoris asperi; alterum molle, lenius odore et fere algae; tertium candidioris vermiculi; quartum pumicosius spongeae putri simile. Paene purpureum quod aptimum; hoc et Milesium vocatur, quo candidius autem, hoc minus probabile est. Vis eorum ut exulcerent, purgent. Usus tostis et sine oleo. Mire lepras lichenas lentigines tollunt cum lupino et sulpuris duobus obolis. Alcyoneo utuntur et ad oculorum cicatrices.

> *Alcyoneum* is found in the sea, from the nests of the alcyon and the ceyx, as some suggest; from the refuse from the congealing of sea-foam, as others suggest; from the slime or, so to speak, 'fluff' of the sea, as others suggest. There are four kinds of it: similar to ashes, dense, of a pungent smell; another soft, milder in smell and like seaweed; the third like a whitish worm; the fourth like pumice, resembling rotting sponge. The best is almost purple; this is also called Milesian, while the whiter it is, the less valuable. Their property is to ulcerate and to cleanse when used. It is dried and applied without oil. With lupins and two *oboli* of sulphur it will miraculously remove leprous sores, lumps and freckles. *Alcyoneum* is also used for scars on the eyes.

Dioscorides (5.118) lists five categories:

> τοῦ δὲ ἀλκυονίου πέντε γνωστέον εἴδη ὑπάρχειν· τὸ μὲν γάρ πυκνόν τέ ἐστι καὶ τῷ ῥυθμῷ σπογγῶδες καὶ βαρύ, ἔτι δὲ βρωμῶδες καὶ ἰχθύος ὄζον, ὃ δὴ πλεῖστον ἐπὶ τῶν ἠιόνων εὑρίσκεται. τὸ δὲ ἑξῆς κατὰ μὲν τὸ σχῆμα πτερυγίῳ ὀφθαλμικῷ ἢ σπόγγῳ ἔοικε, κοῦφον δέ ἐστι καὶ πολύκενον καὶ φυκώδη ἀποφορὰν ἔχον. τὸ δὲ τρίτον σκωληκοειδὲς ὑπάρχει τῷ τύπῳ, καὶ τῇ χρόᾳ

ἐμπόρφυρον, ὅ τινες Μιλήσιον καλοῦσι. τὸ τέταρτον δὲ ἐρίοις οἰσυπηροῖς ὅμοιον, πολύκενον, κοῦφον. τὸ δὲ πέμπτον ἔοικε μὲν κατὰ τὸ σχῆμα μύκητι, ἄνοσμον δέ ἐστι καὶ τραχὺ ἔνδοθεν, κισήρει κατά τι ἐοικός, ἔξωθεν δὲ λεῖον, δριμύ, <ὅ>· πλεῖστον ἐν τῇ Προποντίδι κατὰ τὴν καλουμένην Βέσβικον νῆσον γεννᾶται, ὃ ἐπιχωρίως ἁλὸς ἄχνην καλοῦσι. τούτων τὸ μὲν πρῶτον καὶ δεύτερον εἰς σμήγματα παραλαμβάνεται γυναικῶν, καὶ πρὸς φακούς, λειχῆνάς τε καὶ λέπρας καὶ ἀλφοὺς καὶ μελανίας καὶ σπίλους τοὺς ἐπὶ τοῦ προσώπου καὶ τοῦ λοιποῦ σώματος. τὸ δὲ τρίτον εὐθετεῖ πρὸς δυσουροῦντας καὶ ἀμμώδη συλλέγοντας ἐν τῇ κύστει νεφριτικούς, πρὸς ὕδρωπας, σπλῆνας. καὲν δὲ καὶ καταχρισθὲν σὺν οἴνῳ ἀλωπεκίας θεραπεύει. τὸ δὲ ὕστατον ὀδόντας λευκαίνειν δύναται· παραλαμβάνεται δὲ καὶ εἰς ἄλλα σμήγματα καὶ ψίλωθρα μισγόμενον ἁλσί. καῦσαι δὲ βουλόμενός τι τούτων εἰς ὠμὴν χύτραν ἔμβαλε καὶ περιαλείψας τὸ στόμα αὐτῆς πηλῷ δὸς εἰς κάμινον· ὅταν δὲ ὀπτηθῇ ὁ κέραμος αὐτῆς, ἀνελόμενος ἀπόθου καὶ χρῶ. πλύνεται δὲ ὡς ἡ καδμεία.

One must know, in fact, there are five types of *alcyoneum*. One is thick, sponge-like in shape and dense; it also stinks, smelling of fish; it is found in the largest quantities on the seashore. The next is similar in shape to a membrane from the eye's inner-corner or a sponge; it is light and porous and emits a seaweed-like smell. The third is in the shape of a worm, in fact, and coloured like red dye, which some call Milesian. The fourth is like greasy wool, very porous and light. The fifth is like a mushroom in shape; it is without smell, jagged inside, like pumice, but on the outside it is smooth and sharp; much of it is to be found in Propontis around the island called Besbicos, where the locals call it sea-foam. Of these, the first and the second are used as cleansers for women, and for spots on the body, lichen-like eruptions on the skin, leprosies, dull-white leprosies, black spots, blemishes on the face and the rest of the body. The third is suitable for those with difficult urination and for those with kidney disease who collect gravelly substances in their bladders, for those with fluid retention, and for the spleen. Burned and applied with wine, it treats bald spots. The last has the capacity to whiten teeth and is also used for other cleansers and depilatories when mixed with salt. If you wish to burn any of this, place it into an unbaked clay pot and, having luted the mouth of the pot with clay, put it into an oven. When it is heated; remove it, store and use. It is washed like calamine.

Both Pliny and Dioscorides describe the substance as coming from, or as associated with, the sea. Both list categories that overlap, indicative of a common source, most likely Sextius Niger (Scarborough 2008). Despite ancient (and some modern) uncertainties, *alcyonea* are in fact various types of soft corals (also known as 'bastard' corals or sponges) belonging to the *Alcyoniidae* family; cf. the entry on 'alkuoneion' in Keyser and Irby-Massie (2009). Owing to the plentiful number of *genera* and species, which includes different shapes, sizes, textures and chemical compositions, scholars such as Pliny and Dioscorides were correct in listing the various 'types'. The use of soft corals in pharmaceuticals and cosmeceuticals is increasing in line with research that has proven, for example, antibacterial and anti-inflammatory properties of various species. The ancients were aware of the cleansing qualities of *alcyonea* (cf. also the *Greek Medical Papyri*, cf. Hanson (2009) on the illustrated 'Herbal' from Tebtunis). Pliny mentions that the product is subject to a drying process and Dioscorides notes that it could be heated and then stored for future use (the incineration process producing ammonium carbonate; cf. above p. 64 on hartshorn).

Ovid's interpretation comes from his familiarity with myths and words connected with the kingfisher, which blurs the meaning of the substance. For example, the meaning of the word *alkuōn* in Greek is 'kingfisher' and *alcyonea* in Latin etymologizes its connection with Alcyone. The latter was the daughter of Aeolus (god of the winds) and either Enarete (a mortal) or Aegiale (daughter of Helios), and the wife of Ceyx. Alcyone's story is told in *Met.* 11.410–748: she and her husband arrogantly compared themselves to Juno and Jupiter, respectively, and were punished; Ceyx was drowned in a storm, Alcyone leapt into the sea after him and both were transformed into kingfishers. During winter each year, Aeolus calmed the seas for seven days so Alcyone could make her nest and lay her eggs, hence the phrase 'halcyon days'. Such intertwining of mythology and etymology, with the resultant confusions, has clearly led to Ovid's location of the substance as coming from the kingfisher's nest.

## Lines 83–90 – Recipe 4

At *ll.*83–84 Ovid notes the use of incense in the veneration of gods and angry divine forces, which, as Rosati (1985: 78) comments, sets up an elegant formula of transition to the recipe that follows (*ll.*85ff.). On the use of incense to worship, thank and placate the gods and other divine forces, cf. Scheid (2007);

cf. also Potter (2002) on the use of scent in Rome. Noteworthy also is Ovid's promise of incense to thank the gods if they heed his prayers and save Corinna, suffering from the aftermath of an abortion at *Am.* 2.13.24.

*Ingredients:*
4 oz (109 g) frankincense
4 oz (109 g) natron
¾ cube of gum
1 small cube of myrrh
Honey

*Method:*
Step i: Mix incense with natron
Step ii: Divide the mixture into three exact weighted measures
Step iii: Add the stripped gum less a quarter with myrrh
Step iv: Blend the mixture and sift
Step v: Press the powder together with an infusion of honey

(i) Frankincense (*tus*). In most Latin sources it is difficult to distinguish between incense per se and frankincense as the word most often used for both is *tus* and usually designates frankincense. Frankincense, a gum in the form of large 'tears' from the *Boswellia sacra* tree, was one of the most prized luxury items in antiquity. Pliny (12.51–65) mentions it originated from, and its trade once dominated by, the Minaei (tribes from modern-day Yemen in south-west Arabia). At 12.63 he discusses the changes to the regional domination of the trade in frankincense with the collapse of the Minaei and describes the trade routes and various bureaucratic and financial aspects of importing the highly prized product from Arabia. For an excellent overview of the Arabian spice trade in antiquity, cf. Ben-Yehoshua et al (2012: 10–19).

Frankincense has long been recognized as having 'antibacterial, antibiotic, antifungal, and antiseptic properties ... The *Boswellia* resin is nontoxic to humans and can be applied externally, in combination with other products or alone.' (Ben-Yehoshua et al 2012: 34). In addition to its various uses in ancient and modern medicines, including holistic therapies, the *Boswellia* resin (in powered form) has been used in skin treatments and beautification therapies for thousands of years, treating 'signs of aging, such as wrinkles, skin sagging, dark spots, skin infections, skin irritation, cuts, scarring, acne, cold sores, chapped lips, and varicose veins' (Ibid. 37). Theophrastus (*Enquiry into Plants* 9.11) recommends frankincense mixtures for sores. Celsus recommends frankincense mixtures for cleansing the skin (5.5) and also for effective emollients (5.17). Dioscorides (1.68) cites a plethora of ailments (wounds, ulcerated cavities, warts, eruptions on the face) treated with frankincense recipes and prescribes a mixture of frankincense and soda for a skin cleanser and dandruff remedy; cf. also Miller and Morris (1988: 78–80, 298–304) and, especially, Majno (1975: 207–219).

(ii) Natron (*natrum*), recalling *nitri spuma rubentis* of l.73, is identified as sodium carbonate. Rosati (1985: 79) suggests that the idea behind this line, with the use of 'natron' and the verb *radere* ('to scrape', 'to shave', 'to smooth'), suggests a process that soothes the skin while thoroughly cleansing it. For comment on *radere* and the alternative manuscript reading, cf. p. 138.

(iii) Gum (*gummi* = *cummi*); cf. above p. 65.

(iv) Myrrh (*myrra*), as observed by Riddle (1997: 51), 'was known to Greek mythology before it appeared in Greek medical records' and Ovid includes the aetiology of myrrh in *Met.* 10.298–502. Like many of the tales in the *Metamorphoses*, this one is full of taboo and dire punishments: Myrrha, the daughter of King Cinyras of Assyria, lusted after her father (Ovid blames the Furies) and desires to make love to him. Aided by her nurse, she eventually finds a way to seduce Cinyras in the darkness of night, and for several days, in anonymity, she visits her father and inevitably conceives a child. On Cinyras's discovery of her identity, Myrrha is forced to flee. Tired, heavily pregnant and having walked for months through Arabia, she pleads with the gods to release her, which they do, transforming her into the myrrh tree (*Commiphora myrrha*) while her unborn son, born from bark and foliage, is Adonis. The sap from the tree, myrrh, is known as Myrrha's tears.

Like frankincense, myrrh is a fragrant gum from southern Arabia. In the story, Myrrha walks through the spice regions of Arabia, including the southwest, famous for its frankincense. Like the story, the species *Commiphora myrrha* produces myrrh in the shape of tears. In antiquity, through to modernity, myrrh has played a role in healing; the resin possessing antiinflammatory and antibacterial properties (Ben-Yehoshua et al 2012: 46). Celsus (5.6) lists myrrh as an erodent, indicating that it could be used as an exfoliant as well as a cleanser to remove dead skin cells and more serious facial scurf. Cf. also, Pliny (24.154) on myrrh used to treat sores on the head and face. Dioscorides (1.64) discusses the many uses of myrrh, among them its inclusion in mixtures for facial eruptions and hair loss. In some modern cosmetics, myrrh is used to treat acne and reduce wrinkles. Further on myrrh, cf. Miller and Morris (1988: 82–83, 304–305); Majno (1975: 217–218).

(v) Honey (*mel*). The healing and beautification properties of honey have been discussed above; here honey is used as an emulsifier as in recipes one and two. Ovid mentions a honey infusion (the ingredients are covered with honey and allowed to blend). Such infusions can be with cold or hot honey; cold infusions should, ideally, be left to blend for around two weeks, while hot infusions with warmed honey can be used within a much shorter period of time.

## Lines 91–98 – Recipe 5

*Ingredients:*
0.2 oz (6 g) fennel
0.4 oz (10 g) myrrh
1 handful of dried rose petals
Frankincense
Ammoniac salt
Barley juice

*Method:*
Step i: Add fennel to the myrrh
Step ii: Add dried rose petals with some salt and weigh
Step iii: Weigh the frankincense to equal the rose petals and salt
Step iv: Combine the ingredients
Step v: Infuse the ingredients in barley juice

Some ingredients have already been discussed: myrrh (pp. 76–77), frankincense (pp. 75–76) and barley (pp. 60–61), as well as the infusion process (above). Noteworthy, however, is the inclusion of the adjective *masculum* to describe the frankincense as 'male' at *l*.94. This appellation appears to have originated because of the apparent scrotum-like shape of some forms of the gum that marked it as the finest quality. Further on 'male' and 'female' frankincense, cf. Theophrastus *Enquiry into Plants* 9.2; Pliny 12.61; Dioscorides 1.68.

The remaining ingredients are as follows:

(i) Fennel (*marathus*); cf. Fig. 11. Ovid uses *marathus* from *marathon* rather than *ferula* (the common word for fennel), *Marathōn* (Marathon) being so-named because it was overgrown with fennel. This herb has an extensive history in the Mediterranean, as testified by its inclusion in Linear B (Tablet My 105), possibly as part of a merchant's list; cf. Howe (1958). Pliny mentions it as an ingredient in medical treatments; cf., for example, in a recipe to alleviate oedema or fluid retention (20.43) and in a mixture to relieve joint inflammation (20.195). Dioscorides (3.70) mentions the application of fennel to treat snake and dog bites. All of the plant is useable, although Ovid does not specify a particular part (perhaps the leaf or the seeds as both are still used today in health infusions, including barley water infusions). In modern beauty products it is used primarily as a cleanser (with astringent qualities) and also as an emollient to soften and moisturize the skin.

(ii) Rose (*rosa*). Celsus (5.15) mentions rose petals as an emollient and Pliny (23.94) lists a variety of rose-based remedies (cf., for example, 22.188, 201, 246) as well as the use of rose oil in black hair dye (27.53) and perfume (13.9). Like superior frankincense, rose petals were also a luxury item, particularly in winter, although they were sourced within Italy (cf. *Georgics* 4.119). Rose petals, along with olive oil, beeswax and water constituted Galen's famous cold cream, *ceratum refrigerans Galeni*; a water-in-oil emulsion that continues to be produced in improved formulae. On the measurement of a 'handful', it appears that Ovid is using 'recipe language'; cf. Nicander, who includes 'a handful of fresh berries' in one of his snake-averting salves (*Theriaca* 94) and 'a handful of gypsum' in a draught to alleviate poison (*Alexipharmaca* 43).

(iii) Ammoniac salt is named after the salt obtained near the oracular shrine of Ammon in the Siwah desert. Some suggest that the mineral came from camel dung (and / or urine), which has a high salt content. The excessively dry nature of the dung meant that it could be collected easily and used immediately for fire with the resultant white crystalline deposit a source of ammonium chloride; cf. Majno (1975: 139, 487n282) who discusses the various theories behind its origins. It is likely that Ovid is referring to a common form of rock

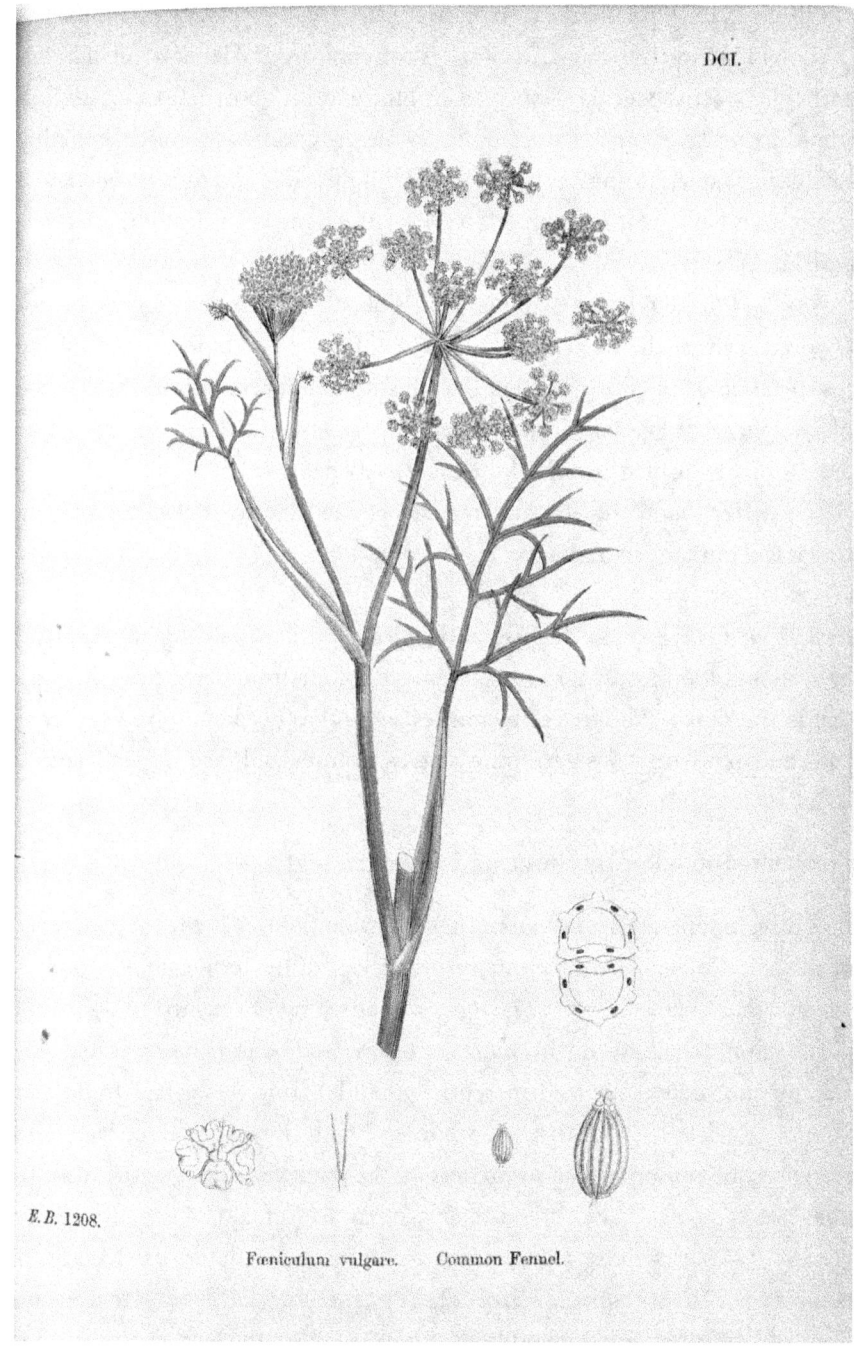

**Fig. 11** Fennel (*Foeniculum vulgare*).

salt given the 'Egyptian' label for prestige purposes because it resembled the salt obtained from the shrine. Rock salt is common around igneous formations, particularly active volcanoes such as Mt Etna and Mt Vesuvius, occurring as a white, crusty layer on the volcanic fumarole. Ammonium chloride is highly soluble in water, forming a solution that is mildly acidic and thus excellent as a cleanser and exfoliant for skin (cf. p. 64 for the same beautification effects as hartshorn).

Rosati (1985: 80) states that it is impossible to tell from the recipe whether Ovid means that the frankincense should equal the combined weight of the rose petals and the salt, or whether the salt and frankincense should each equal the weight of the petals. It seems most sensible to interpret the recipe as indicating the former in view of the excessively light weight of petals.

(iv) Barley (*hordeum*). The barley is steeped in water to make barley water, which will bind the ingredients.

At *ll*.97–98 Ovid explains the use of the *medicamen*, namely it is to be spread over one's *vultus* ('features') and will remove 'colour' from the entire *os* ('face'); that is, the skin will be free of blemishes. *vultus* has been employed earlier at *l*.46 and *l*.67 where it has been translated as 'features' and 'face' respectively.

## Lines 99–100 – Poppy rouge and a broken text

Like roses, poppies provide natural rouge. Stewart (2007: 42) cites several types of rouge in Rome: *faex* (quite often wine dregs, but the term can also imply a generic 'muck'; cf. below p. 122); *morum* (consisting of crushed mulberries); *purpurissum* (chalk dyed with *murex*); *rubrica* (red ochre). Stewart (Ibid. 43) also mentions *cinnabar* (red mercuric sulphide) from Spain and India and *minium* (red lead), noting that 'like white lead, both cinnabar and red lead were known to be poisonous, an awareness of the dangers, among some at least, does not appear to have curbed their general use' (cf. also, *Rem.* 351). Pliny (28.184–185) lists more exotic rouges such as bull's dung, particularly if combined with *crocodilea* or 'crocodile' dung. *crocodilea* likely refers to the dung of a lizard or land 'crocodile'; cf. Pliny 28.28 (on the land 'crocodile' that eats fragrant flowers and produces the sweet-smelling substance, *crocodilea*); cf. also Galen 12.47–48 Kühn 1826; 12.308 Kühn 1826. Olson (2009: 297) notes an alternative identification, namely *crocodilea* as 'an Egyptian code-word for "Ethiopian soil"' that was 'a particular earth found beyond Upper Egypt'. Olson also mentions Lemnian and Samian 'earths' that were highly prized for skin preparations, and references Betz's adoption of 'Ethiopian soil' for *crocodilea* in his edition of *Greek Magical Papyri* XII.401–444 (168). On the possibility of Ovid referring to the latter as a complexion lightener at *AA* 3.270, cf. Hendry (1995); Gibson (2003: 206).

Green (1979: 390) comments on the benefits of poppies for healthy skin: 'It has been shown that certain essential fatty acids in poppy seeds, especially some isomers of linolenic acid, are effective against eczema, dry skin, and scalp disease.' He also notes the benefits of rubbing one's face with a mixture that includes cold water: 'Cold water and rubbing are highly beneficial for the complexion, producing a healthy glow.'

## 2

# *Amores* 1.14

### Latin text

Dicebam 'medicare tuos desiste capillos';
    tingere quam possis, iam tibi nulla coma est.
At si passa fores, quid erat spatiosius illis?
    Contigerant imum qua patet usque latus.
Quid, quod erant tenues et quos ornare timeres,      5
    vela colorati qualia Seres habent,
vel pede quod gracili deducit aranea filum,
    cum leve deserta sub trabe nectit opus?
Nec tamen ater erat, nec erat tamen aureus ille
    sed, quamvis neuter, mixtus uterque color,      10
qualem clivosae madidis in vallibus Idae
    ardua derepto cortice cedrus habet.
Adde, quod et dociles et centum flexibus apti
    et tibi nullius causa doloris erant.
Non acus abrupit, non vallum pectinis illos;      15
    ornatrix tuto corpore semper erat;
ante meos saepe est oculos ornata nec umquam
    bracchia derepta saucia fecit acu.
Saepe etiam nondum digestis mane capillis
    purpureo iacuit semisupina toro;      20
tum quoque erat neglecta decens, ut Thracia Bacche,
    cum temere in viridi gramine lassa iacet.
Cum graciles essent tamen et lanuginis instar,
    heu, mala vexatae quanta tulere comae!

Quam se praebuerunt ferro patienter et igni, 25
 ut fieret torto nexilis orbe sinus!
Clamabam 'scelus est istos, scelus, urere crines.
 Sponte decent: capiti, ferrea, parce tuo.
Vim procul hinc remove: non est, qui debeat uri;
 erudit admotas ipse capillus acus' 30
Formosae periere comae, quas vellet Apollo,
 quas vellet capiti Bacchus inesse suo;
illis contulerim, quas quondam nuda Dione
 pingitur umenti sustinuisse manu.
Quid male dispositos quereris periisse capillos? 35
 Quid speculum maesta ponis inepta manu?
Non bene consuetis a te spectaris ocellis:
 ut placeas, debes immemor esse tui.
Non te cantatae laeserunt paelicis herbae,
 non anus Haemonia perfida lavit aqua, 40
nec tibi vis morbi nocuit (procul omen abesto),
 nec minuit densas invida lingua comas.
Facta manu culpaque tua dispendia sentis;
 ipsa dabas capiti mixta venena tuo.
Nunc tibi captivos mittet Germania crines; 45
 tuta triumphatae munere gentis eris.
O quam saepe comas aliquo mirante rubebis
 et dices 'empta nunc ego merce probor.
nescioquam pro me laudat nunc iste Sygambram;
 fama tamen memini cum fuit ista mea.' 50
Me miserum! Lacrimas male continet oraque dextra
 protegit ingenuas picta rubore genas;
sustinet antiquos gremio spectatque capillos,
 ei mihi, non illo munera digna loco.
Collige cum vultu mentem: reparabile damnum est; 55
 postmodo nativa conspiciere coma.

## Translation

I was constantly saying 'Desist from treating your locks';
   now there is not a tress left for you to dye.
Ah, but if you had allowed it, what was more abundant than those locks?
   They had reached down to your side as far as it extends.
What of the fact that they were finely textured and the kind you would
   fear to adorn, like the cloth the coloured Chinese have,       5
or the thread the spider spins with delicate foot,
   when it weaves its gossamer work beneath an abandoned beam?
Yet its colour was neither black, yet neither was it gold
   but, although neither of the two, combined both,       10
like the lofty cedar in the moist valleys of steep Ida
   possesses when stripped of its bark.
Moreover, they were compliant and adaptable to infinite styles
   and to you not a cause of anger.
The hairpin did not break them, nor the teeth of the comb;       15
   the hairdresser's body was always safe;
often was she adorned before my eyes but never
   has she caused wounded arms by snatching at a hairpin.
Often as well with her locks not yet arranged in the early morning
   she would lie half-reclining on her purple bed;       20
then also was she becoming in her neglect, like a Thracian Bacchant,
   when carelessly she sprawls exhausted on the lush grass.
But while finely textured and like down,
   alas, what great misfortunes those tortured tresses endured!
How patiently they offered themselves up to steel and fire,       25
   so that a wavy appearance from shaped coils could be produced!
I used to shout 'It is a crime, a crime, to scorch those hairs.
   They are naturally becoming: be sparing of your head, girl-of-iron.
Violence begone far from here: your hair is not the kind to be scorched;
   the lock itself educates the hairpins attached to it'.       30
The beautiful tresses have perished, which Apollo would want,
   which Bacchus would want upon his own head;

I could compare them to those which naked Dione
    in her portrait held up with dripping hand.
Why do you complain at the loss of these badly styled locks?    35
    Why do you, foolish one, set aside your mirror with sorrowful hand?
It is not good for you to look at yourself with your usual stare:
    in order to please yourself, try to be forgetful of yourself.
The charmed herbs of a rival have not harmed you,
    a treacherous old hag has not bathed you in Haemonian water,    40
nor has the violence of a disease harmed you (let such an ill be far away),
    nor has an envious tongue thinned your thick tresses.
You are suffering the results of your own handiwork and your own mistakes;
    you blended and applied the poisons to your own head.
Now to you will Germany send captive hair;    45
    safe will you be via the gift of a conquered people.
O how often you will blush when people marvel at your tresses
    and you will say 'Because of something purchased I am now admired.
Now he is praising an unknown Sygambrian woman instead of me;
    yet I remember when such glory was entirely my own'.    50
Wretched me! She can barely hold back tears and she covers her features
    with her right hand, staining her tender cheeks with a blush;
she holds her former locks in her lap and gazes upon them,
    ah me, gifts not worthy of that place.
Compose your mind along with your face: the damage is reparable:    55
    soon you will be noticed for your natural tresses.

## Commentary

In this evocative scene of the day in the life of the *amator* of the *Amores*, Ovid describes a cosmetic emergency. Most scholars identify the *puella* of the poem as Corinna, Ovid's 'go-to' girl when a consistent lover is required for a sense of cohesion in the collection, or when one is needed to act in a particular *mise en scène* that expresses a particular erotic situation (cf. *Am.* 1.5, 1.11, 2.6, 2.8, 2.11, 2.12, 2.13, 2.17, 2.19, 3.1, 3.7, 3.12).

Corinna makes her formal, named entrance at *Am.* 1.5, typifying the beautiful *meretrix*, wearing a *tunica* (literally an undergarment) – not a *palla* or *stola* – with cascading hair, unrestrained by *vittae*. At *Am.* 2.19.46 she is an *uxor* ('wife') with a *maritus* (2.19.57). The contradictions are problematic to say the least (cf. above p. 38 n. 17) and may well suggest that Corinna is, ultimately, a life-like fake, usefully inserted where needed (cf. McKeown 1: 19–24; Miller 2013).

Despite a reading of the *Amores* that prejudices each elegy as narratological 'snapshots' that ultimately ask the reader to participate in imagining and making their own interpretative connections between the poems (cf. Salzman-Mitchell 2008), there are obvious themes that filter throughout it (cf. above pp. 28–29). The elegiac lover's interest in cosmetics is one of these themes and here, in keeping with the traditional voice of the *amator*, Ovid relinquishes his usual supportive stance on female adornment. He does so, not because he is being moralistic, but because cosmetics in this instance have not enhanced natural beauty but ruined it.

## Lines 1–2 – I was constantly saying . . .

Ovid inserts himself as the dominant voice in this melodrama with the opening verb *dicebam* ('I was constantly saying'). The verb indicates that Corinna's misfortune, and the actions of which she was guilty, are interpreted – judged – by him. The topic of Corinna's exceedingly bad hair day is immediately addressed and thus, for the remainder of the poem, Ovid can reflect on it from a variety of angles. He first reminds Corinna that he had warned her to desist from dyeing her hair (the verb *medicare* to describe the process of dyeing is discussed above, p. 49), and then proceeds to address the catastrophic result of chemical colouring – baldness – of which she would be well aware.

On the variety of dyes on the Roman market, Stewart (2007: 90) comments: 'The sheer number of products for which we have a record suggests that hair dye, in a range of colours, was much in demand.' While blonde was the shade most often associated with the hair of courtesans and prostitutes in general, some gods were also blond. Stewart (Ibid. 44) observes that Aurora, Ceres, Apollo and Mercury 'traditionally had blonde hair' and this divine ideal of paleness, of both skin and hair, was regarded as aesthetically pleasing to the Romans. As the Italians did not tend to be natural blondes, there were various formulae for lightening and bleaching hair.

As Olson (2008a: 72) notes, most of the extant sources that provide recipes for hair dye come from the genre of technical or scientific / medical writing. Pliny provides numerous recipes, most of them for black hair dye: elderberries (16.180); bitter vetch (22.153); leeches rotted in red wine for forty days (32.67); a form of bituminous earth called *ampelitis* – also for a dark eyelash tint (35.194); St John's wort, orchids and Greek valerian boiled down in oil (26.164). For blonde or flaxen hair he recommends nightshade juice (26.164). He also lists ingredients for red / golden hair dye made from young walnuts (15.87) and a German formula of ash (preferably from beechwood, according to d'Ambrosio 2001: 17) and suet called *sapo* (28.191). Olson (2008a: 73) suggests that *sapo* may be the cosmetic culprit behind the disaster of *Am.* 1.14; a possibility perhaps further alluded to by Ovid's arboreal imagery (*ll.*9–12), which may be an otiose reference to the tree ash used in the recipe.

As the expert on female *cultus*, Ovid ensures he demonstrates the various terms for hair:

(i) The plural *capilli* (*l.*1) is translated as 'locks'. The noun is repeated in both singular and plural at *l.*19, *l.*30, *l.*35, *l.*53; cf. also *Med.* 19; *AA* 3.133, 145 and *AA* 3.235.

(ii) The plural *crines*, translated as the collective 'hair' at *l.*27 and *l.*45; cf. also *AA* 3.141, 243.

(iii) The frequent noun *coma* is translated as 'tress'. It is repeated in both singular and plural at *l.*24, *l.*31, *l.*42, *l.*47, *l.*56; cf. also *Med.* l.29 and *AA* 3.238, 246. The similarity in meaning between *coma* and *capillus* is succinctly addressed by McKeown (2: 365), who notes that just as *tingere* may be used synonymously with *medicare*, so may *coma* with *capillus*. To maintain the similarity while denoting the two discrete Latin terms, *coma* = 'tress' and *capillus* = 'lock' throughout the translations, with some exceptions: *AA* 3.153 ('hair' is contextually apt for *coma*), *AA* 3.161 (*capilli* is rendered as 'hairs' to suit the topic of men's hair), *AA* 1.505 (*capillus* = 'hair') and also *AA* 1.518 (*coma* = 'hair').

## Lines 3–12 – Three similes

The erotic homage to Corinna's hair begins at *l*.4 with the designation of the part of the body – the side – used to denote its length. The beauty of Corinna's hair, and the image of it caressing her body, reiterate the connections between hair, beauty and sexual appeal. According to Bartman (2001:1): 'In ancient Rome hair was a major determinant of a woman's physical attractiveness' and 'women typically had more "symbolic capital" invested in their hair than men did, and few protested the attention paid to it.' (Ibid. 3–4). The powerful gendered and social symbolisms associated with women's hair emphatically underscore the disastrous implications of Corinna's baldness.

Ovid eulogizes Corinna's hair in three evocative similes:

(i) Chinese cloth. A reference to antiquity's most superior silk. While at this stage most Romans were probably ignorant of why Chinese silk was superior, it is interesting to note the reason, in order to better understand Ovid's reference to it. Made from the *Bombyx mori* moth species by boiling cocoons before the moths escape, the Chinese could produce continuous filaments without the need to spin the thread. In contrast, the silk in Asia Minor and India was harvested after the moth had eaten through the cocoon, which resulted in a poorer quality of silk because the threads were broken and had to be (re)woven. The reference to Chinese silk thus illustrates the superior nature of Corinna's hair by suggesting its delicacy and, in particular, its beautiful long strands. Additionally, the noun *vela*, which also means 'sails' and other billowy items, is suggestive of the hair's buoyancy and evokes a sense of its movement.

(ii) The spider's web. The imagery of Chinese silk is an apt simile to precede and match the spider's web. Comparing Corinna's hair to the spider's web is not merely another testimony to its loveliness, but also its fine texture. Similar to the silks of moth and spider, human hair cannot withstand heavy-handed 'improvement'; like spilling strong dyes on precious silk, or applying a curling iron to a web, 'beautifying' Corinna's locks with harsh products and heated steel is destined to ruin it.

(iii) The lofty cedar, stripped of bark. Ovid's tree, an object of beauty and awe, is from the moist valleys of Ida, a high mountain in Phrygia near Troy.

While the simile is essentially one that compares the colour of the locks to the cedar, the valley, by implication, also becomes associated with the body of the woman. Hardie (2002: 58) has discussed Ovidian equations between landscape and the female body; in *Am.* 2.16, for example, 'the thought of a rich grassy growth overshadowing moist places brings the poet up against the realization that he is far from the body of the beloved.' He also cites *Met.* 4.300–301 and 'the vaginal image of Salmacis' pool fringed with grass' (58n65); cf. also Keith (2009); Segal (1969); Hinds (2002).

Like the confusion over the different types of silk, there was confusion over the identifications of trees in antiquity. In fact, as Boyd (1997: 120–121) points out, Ovid's reference to *cedrus* ('cedar') is wrong and the tree best suited to his description is the *fraxinus* ('mountain ash'), which in contrast to the cedar, actually grows near Troy. Both trees were misidentified in antiquity because of the very characteristic to which Ovid refers, namely the colour of their trunks; that is, stripped of its outer bark, cedar possesses the auburn colour of ash. Pliny (16.62) explains that people were often tricked into buying stripped cedar, believing it to be ash. Boyd (1997: 121) therefore suggests that the tree of *Am.* 1.14 'appears to be a conflation based on ... traditional confusion; the reference to Ida thus becomes not just an otiose descriptive detail but a casual index of Ovid's learning' (cf. also Papaioannou 2006: 46). In other words, Ovid was actually cognizant of the intricacies of dendrology (and maybe the cunning scam in the ash and cedar market) and is being clever. To push this interpretation further, one may argue that he chose the image – complete with its inherent dissimulations – as a comment on humankind's interference in nature and its associated deceptions (pretending that he *himself* is mistaken). To exhaust this interpretive potential further by considering a connection to *cultus* and trickery, the metaphoric association between hair and tree is in order. Such a simile would usually compare tresses to leaves but Ovid compares colour to trunk (a trunk stripped bare). While it has been suggested that the image plays with both scientific knowledge and ignorance, it is also evocative of a 'bark-less' tree and a 'hair-less' head. As the greedy timber merchants interfere in nature to transform cedar into ash, Corinna interferes in nature to transform hair colour. Like the cedar, Corinna too has lost her covering, but, as Ovid goes on to advise her, she can always protect her stripped head with a wig (a man-made bark covering).

## Lines 13–18 – Roman hairdressing

On the topic of the flexibility of the locks, Ovid points out to Corinna that they were pliant enough to furnish 'infinite stylings'. He specifies several components of a woman's hair-styling process:

(i) Multiple styles. Long hair was a requisite for Roman women in order to achieve ornate and varied styles. Bartman (2001: 12) notes that there was a variety of hair cosmetics available to achieve a particular coiffure without the addition of hair pieces; these included waxes (such as gum arabic) and creams that could be used with a curling iron. Further on Ovid's reference to multiple styles, cf. *Am.* 2.8.1 and *AA* 3.135–160 (below, pp. 110–112).

(ii) Hairpin (*acus*). The use of the hairpin (or bodkin) was both practical and ornamental. Hairpins were fashioned from wood, bone, crystal and metals and were variously decorated with both simple and intricate designs. Olson (2008a: 75) describes hairpins 'tipped with glass beads or pendants, decorated heads, or carved ends in the shape of hands, vases, animals, or mythological figures' and even 'adorned women'. On hairpins, Stephens (2008: 115) writes:

> [They] depend on *isometrics* to hold the hair in place: the hair must be coiled or twisted tightly so that, once the hair bodkin is inserted, the push of the hair against each end of the hair bodkin is balanced by a pull along the middle of the shaft. If there is too little isometric tension, the hair bodkin will fall out and the hair will collapse. Hair bodkins can easily support tight buns and twists with a pleasing decorative effect but, because of their reliance on stress and tension, they have major limitations if they are expected to be the sole support of a hairstyle.

Thus, for the exceedingly intricate styles of the imperial age, Stephens argues that the Roman hairdresser most likely employed a needle-and-thread to literally stitch braids of hair into place.

(iii) Comb (*pecten*). Combs were usually made of wood or bone. Double-sided H-shaped combs had a coarse side for detangling, general grooming and keeping the hair in place (like a hairpin), and a fine side for more intricate styling, delousing and other hygiene procedures. Cf. Figs 3 and 5 (the comb is to the right of the mirror).

(iv) The hairdresser (*ornatrix*). In most cases the hairdresser was a female slave in the household. Like the *tractatrix* ('beautician') and *unctrix* ('masseuse' and 'anointer'), the hairdresser belonged to a category of slaves trained in a specific skill. Freedwomen were also hairdressers, working in public venues; cf. Treggiari (1976); cf. also Martial 2.17 on a female barber in the Subura; cf. *AA* 3.239ff.

At *ll*.16–18 Ovid mentions that Corinna did not have to resort to attacks on her hairdresser (so manageable were her locks). This indicates, as attested by other poets, that violence against personal slaves such as *ornatrices* was not uncommon. On this topic, cf. Martial 2.66 on Lalage who assaults her hairdresser with a mirror and Juvenal's hairdressing scene in 6.487–505 that features an *ornatrix*, Psecas, who is attacked by her mistress. Both Corinna and Ovid share 'intimate' relationships with Corinna's hairdressers – obviously treating them as slaves – but experiencing 'relationships' with them all the same. The intense and complex intersubjectivity of such relations is evidenced in *Am.* 1.11, where Ovid addresses Nape, a hairdresser described as *docta* ('skilled'), revealing that she is his messenger, taking his communications to Corinna and monitoring her responses. In *Am.* 2.7 Corinna suspects Ovid has slept with her hairdresser, Cypassis – which he denies – but in *Am.* 2.8, in an address to *fusca Cypassis* ('dark Cypassis'), he reveals the truth behind the allegation. Such intimacies, though always controlled by the asymmetries of power, are also evident in what appear to be more genuinely positive expressions of fondness on the part of the master or mistress; cf. the inscription set up by Pieris to her *ornatrix*, Gnome, in 2 BC (*Corpus Inscriptionum Latinarum* 6.9730).

## Lines 19–22 – Hair *au naturel*

The poet returns to his homage and reveals his preference when it comes to Corinna's hairstyle; he likes it natural and dishevelled. The image suggests an unadorned state antithetical to *cultus* (but cf., below *AA* 3.153–154). As the colour of her hair is compared to cedar stripped of its bark in a moist valley, the image of her on her bed evokes the simile of the Bacchant on lush grass. As the valley is damp, the grass is luxuriant; both comparisons suggestive of the sensual softness and moisture of nature and the women associated with it. The wild nature of the Bacchants, experiencing the divine intoxication of the god and thus liberated from social conventions, is regularly symbolized by their unbound hair. In Catullus 64.61–68 Ariadne stands on the shoreline like a statue of a Bacchant, hair unkempt and semi-naked and in Propertius 1.3.1–8 the poet compares the sleeping Cynthia to an exhausted Bacchant (also to Ariadne). Elsewhere, Ovid includes what Gibson (2003: 222) defines as 'the "bacchant" look'; cf. *Am.* 1.9.37–38 on Agamemnon who, on seeing Cassandra, like a Trojan Maenad with flowing hair, becomes enamoured; *AA* 1.527–541 on Ariadne who, veiled by a loose robe, barefoot, with her yellow hair unbound, is unknowingly ready for Bacchus, who arrives with Bacchants, also with flowing hair; cf. also *AA* 3.157ff. (p. 112) and also *ll.*783ff.

## Lines 23–30 – The *calamistrum*

Ovid evokes the locks further, vividly personifying each one as if it were an individual slave subjected to the proverbial torture of steel and fire in the form of the curling iron. At *l.*25 he refers to, but does not name, the curling iron (*calamistrum*). The specific form of the *calamistrum* in Rome is contested. Olson (2008b: 73) states that it came in two parts: a hollow metal cylinder with a solid metal cylinder inside. The process involved heating the outer cylinders in a fire, wrapping strands of hair around the solid cylinders and placing them inside the hot containers. Stephens argues that it took the form of a long, thin needle, much like the *acus* or hairpin, with a tapered shape that was heated. Stephens cites the stele of the mason, P. Ferrarius Hermes (*Corpus Inscriptionum Latinarum* 11.1471), which shows various items of measurement as well as adornment, including an object resembling her description of the *calamistrum* (cf. Fig. 6, the *calamistrum* is to the right of the mirror, under the comb). Additionally, she cites Isidorus *Etymologiae* 20.13:

> Calamistrum acus est quae calefacta et adhibita calefacit et intorquet capillos. Unde et calamistrati appellantur qui comam torquent.

> The *calamistrum* is a needle (*acus*) that, when heated and applied, heats and curls hair. Those who curl their hair are thereby called 'curled' (*calamistrati*).

Other identifications are based on various modern curling irons and interpretations of archaeological finds, particularly from Pompeii. Despite the debate, whatever implement constituted the *calamistrum*, the damage to the hair could be severe, particularly if the heating process was intense, the practice a regular one and the hair already damaged by colourants.

## Lines 31–34 – Divinely beautiful locks

The hair was so beautiful, even Apollo and Bacchus would want to have it as their own. Both of these gods are known for their flowing locks; cf. especially the imagery of Apollo's hair, never to be shorn, in *Met.* 1.564. Ovid extends his praise of the hair by comparing it to the famous painting of Venus Anadyomene by Apelles (*fl.* fourth century BC), which was consecrated by Augustus in honour of his adoptive father, Caesar, and displayed in the Temple of the Divine Julius in the Roman forum (cf. Pliny 35.36); cf. also *AA* 3.224, 401 and *Tr.* 2.527; Propertius 3.9.11. The Venus Anadyomene became an iconic artistic motif that was replicated in various media from mosaics to sculptures and inscribed gems (on the latter cf. p. 123); cf. also Barsby (1973: 153); Benediktson (1985: 115). Ovid refers to Venus by her alternative name, Dione, the name of her mother; cf. *Fast.* 2.461; 5.309.

## Lines 35–44 – Witchcraft

At *ll.*35–36, the remaining locks are described as having died, recalling the earlier personification of them as tortured slaves. Corinna, having persecuted them until they expire and having thereby rendered herself completely bald, cannot bear to gaze at her reflection. Ovid's 'consolation' takes the rhetorical form of a discussion of witchcraft (*ll.*37–44):

(i) A rival has not resorted to *cantatae herbae* ('charmed herbs') administered by a *perfida anus* ('a treacherous old hag'). Kenney (1958: 58) provides an insightful interpretation of *ll.*39–40, suggesting that, in Ovid's hypothetical situation, an unknown woman arranges for one of Corinna's attendants, 'probably her nurse', to wash her mistress's hair with a poisonous concoction, recalling *Med.* l.37 in which the poet advises women not to trust in grasses or mixtures of juices. The link between poisoned enchantments and cosmetics makes sense of Ovid's idea of 'washing in magic water' (Kenney 1958: 58), further reinforced by Kenney's point that 'cosmetic washes for the hair were in vogue, and some of them must have been very curiously compounded' (citing Pliny 33.109 on a face and hair mixture including lead sulphide). Ovid describes the hypothetical water with the adjective *Haemonia* ('Haemonian'), a poetic name for Thessaly, renowned for its high population of magic practitioners.

(ii) Just as no one has conspired to wash Corinna's hair with a magical potion, there have not been any supernatural forces that have caused the baldness by means of illness. Like other ancient Mediterranean peoples, the Romans believed that malevolent forces could be summoned merely by speaking about something evil or ill-omened. Therefore, phrases such as *procul omen abesto* ('let such an ill be far away') are standard expressions in the context of apotropaic magic; cf. Lateiner (2005: 35–57, especially 47).

(iii) Lastly, an envious tongue has not put a spell on Corinna. The use of the noun *venena* is a clever choice; meaning a spell or potion, but also a poison or a dye, it encapsulates Ovid's images of magical poison as well as the overall theme of the lethal hair colourant. Not administered by a wicked witch on behalf of a malevolent rival, Corinna's misfortune is by her own hands, for she administered the *venena* herself. On magic in antiquity, cf. above pp. 55–57.

## Lines 45–52 – Wigs

Ovid turns to the subject of a suitable wig for Corinna. Olson (2008b: 74) states that there were two types of wigs available: the *capillamentum* ('wig') and the *galerum* ('hairpiece'). In view of Corinna's dilemma, a *capillamentum* would be in order, and it shall be sourced from the captive peoples of Germany. Wigs from Germany were popular and, as the hair tended to be golden and thick, the market was strong. The reference to the Sygambrian woman at *l*.49, whose hair Corinna will purchase, alludes to the Germanic tribe, east of the Lower Danube, known for their long hair and bellicose nature (cf. *On the Spectacles* 3.9 where Martial mentions that they curled their hair in knots). The phrase *captivos crines* ('captured hair'), also used by Martial at 14.26 (cf. Levy 1968), makes a point again about empire and luxury, associating a woman like Corinna with the conquered peoples in two ways: as their imitator as well as their exploiter.

At *AA* 3.163–168 (pp. 112–113), Ovid returns to the subject of women dyeing their hair, referring to 'German herbs', possibly *sapo*, which produce outcomes better than the original colour. He is also positive about wigs and explains that their purchase should not cause a woman to blush (*rubor*). While this is an apparent turnaround, it seems that he is open-minded about dyes and wigs – just not when it comes to Corinna, but this situation is an emergency.

### Lines 53–56 – A blush and some reassurance

Ovid explains that the damage is reparable; Corinna's beautiful hair will soon grow back and she will be noticed once more. The ending maintains the egocentric focus of the poem ('Wretched me!, *l*.51) as well as the light-hearted comedy. Corinna blushes (*l*.52) from embarrassment, not *pudor*, which may reinforce the reading proffered earlier (cf. above pp. 30–31) that suggests she is a cheap version of the heroic, goodly wife, Berenice. If the suggestion is a viable one, perhaps Ovid may be regarded as a not-so-heroic Ptolemy III Euergetes.

# 3

## *Ars Amatoria* 3.101–250

### Latin text

Ordior a cultu: cultis bene Liber ab uvis
 provenit, et culto stat seges alta solo.
Forma dei munus; forma quota quaeque superbit?
 Pars vestrum tali munere magna caret.
Cura dabit faciem; facies neglecta peribit, 105
 Idaliae similis sit licet illa deae.
Corpora si veteres non sic coluere puellae,
 nec veteres cultos sic habuere viros.
Si fuit Andromache tunicas induta valentes,
 quid mirum? Duri militis uxor erat. 110
Scilicet Aiaci coniunx ornata venires,
 cui tegumen septem terga fuere boum!
Simplicitas rudis ante fuit; nunc aurea Roma est
 et domiti magnas possidet orbis opes.
Aspice quae nunc sunt Capitolia, quaeque fuerunt: 115
 alterius dices illa fuisse Iovis.
Curia consilio nunc est dignissima tanto,
 de stipula Tatio regna tenente fuit.
Quae nunc sub Phoebo ducibusque Palatia fulgent,
 quid nisi araturis pascua bubus erant? 120
Prisca iuvent alios, ego me nunc denique natum
 gratulor: haec aetas moribus apta meis,
non quia nunc terrae lentum subducitur aurum
 lectaque diverso litore concha venit,

nec quia decrescunt effosso marmore montes, 125
    nec quia caeruleae mole fugantur aquae,
sed quia cultus adest nec nostros mansit in annos
    rusticitas priscis illa superstes avis.

Vos quoque nec caris aures onerate lapillis,
    quos legit in viridi decolor Indus aqua, 130
nec prodite graves insuto vestibus auro:
    per quas nos petitis, saepe fugatis, opes.
Munditiis capimur: non sint sine lege capilli;
    admotae formam dantque negantque manus.
Nec genus ornatus unum est: quod quamque decebit 135
    eligat et speculum consulat ante suum.
Longa probat facies capitis discrimina puri:
    sic erat ornatis Laodamia comis.
Exiguum summa nodum sibi fronte relinqui,
    ut pateant aures, ora rotunda volunt. 140
Alterius crines umero iactentur utroque:
    talis es adsumpta, Phoebe canore, lyra.
Altera succinctae religetur more Dianae,
    ut solet, attonitas cum petit illa feras.
Huic decet inflatos laxe iacuisse capillos, 145
    illa sit adstrictis impedienda comis.
Hanc placet ornari testudine Cyllenea,
    sustineat similes fluctibus illa sinus.
Sed neque ramosa numerabis in ilice glandes,
    nec quot apes Hybla nec quot in Alpe ferae, 150
nec mihi tot positus numero conprendere fas est:
    adicit ornatus proxima quaeque dies.
Et neglecta decet multas coma: saepe iacere
    hesternam credas, illa repexa modo est.
Ars casum simulet: sic capta vidit ut urbe 155
    Alcides Iolen, 'hanc ego' dixit 'amo'.
Talem te Bacchus Satyris clamantibus 'euhoe'
    sustulit in currus, Cnosi relicta, suos.

O quantum indulget vestro natura decori,
　　quarum sunt multis damna pianda modis! 160
Nos male detegimur, raptique aetate capilli,
　　ut Borea frondes excutiente, cadunt.
Femina canitiem Germanis inficit herbis,
　　et melior vero quaeritur arte color;
femina procedit densissima crinibus emptis 165
　　proque suis alios efficit aere suos.
Nec rubor est emisse: palam venire videmus
　　Herculis ante oculos virgineumque chorum.

Quid de veste loquar? nec vos, segmenta, requiro
　　nec te, quae Tyrio murice, lana, rubes. 170
Cum tot prodierint pretio leviore colores,
　　quis furor est census corpore ferre suos?
Aeris, ecce, color, tum cum sine nubibus aer
　　nec tepidus pluvias concitat auster aquas;
ecce tibi similis, quae quondam Phrixon et Hellen 175
　　diceris Inois eripuisse dolis.
Hic undas imitatur, habet quoque nomen ab undis:
　　crediderim Nymphas hac ego veste tegi;
ille crocum simulat (croceo velatur amictu,
　　roscida luciferos cum dea iungit equos), 180
hic Paphias myrtos, hic purpureas amethystos
　　albentesve rosas Threiciamve gruem.
Nec glandes, Amarylli, tuae, nec amygdala desunt,
　　et sua velleribus nomina cera dedit.
Quot nova terra parit flores, cum vere tepenti 185
　　vitis agit gemmas pigraque fugit hiems,
lana tot aut plures sucos bibit: elige certos,
　　nam non conveniens omnibus omnis erit.
Pulla decent niveas: Briseida pulla decebant;
　　cum rapta est, pulla tum quoque veste fuit. 190
Alba decent fuscas: albis, Cephei, placebas;
　　sic tibi vestitae pressa Seriphos erat.

Quam paene admonui, ne trux caper iret in alas
    neve forent duris aspera crura pilis!
Sed non Caucasea doceo de rupe puellas                           195
    quaeque bibant undas, Myse Caice, tuas.
Quid si praecipiam ne fuscet inertia dentes,
    oraque suscepta mane laventur aqua?
Scitis et inducta candorem quaerere creta;
    sanguine quae vero non rubet, arte rubet.                            200
Arte supercilii confinia nuda repletis
    parvaque sinceras velat aluta genas.
Nec pudor est oculos tenui signare favilla
    vel prope te nato, lucide Cydne, croco.
Est mihi, quo dixi vestrae medicamina formae,                   205
    parvus, sed cura grande, libellus, opus.
Hinc quoque praesidium laesae petitote figurae;
    non est pro vestris ars mea rebus iners.

Non tamen expositas mensa deprendat amator
    pyxidas: ars faciem dissimulata iuvat.                                  210
Quem non offendat toto faex illita vultu,
    cum fluit in tepidos pondere lapsa sinus?
Oesypa quid redolent, quamvis mittatur Athenis
    demptus ab immundo vellere sucus ouis!
Nec coram mixtas cervae sumpsisse medullas                        215
    nec coram dentes defricuisse probem.
Ista dabunt formam, sed erunt deformia visu,
    multaque, dum fiunt turpia, facta placent.
Quae nunc nomen habent operosi signa Myronis,
    pondus iners quondam duraque massa fuit.                       220
Anulus ut fiat, primo colliditur aurum;
    quas geritis vestes, sordida lana fuit.
Cum fieret, lapis asper erat; nunc, nobile signum,
    nuda Venus madidas exprimit imbre comas.
Tu quoque dum coleris, nos te dormire putemus:                 225
    aptius a summa conspiciere manu.

Cur mihi nota tuo causa est candoris in ore?
   Claude forem thalami: quid rude prodis opus?
Multa viros nescire decet; pars maxima rerum
   offendat, si non interiora tegas. 230
Aurea quae splendent ornato signa theatro
   inspice, contemnes: brattea ligna tegit.
Sed neque ad illa licet populo, nisi facta, venire,
   nec nisi summotis forma paranda viris.

At non pectendos coram praebere capillos, 235
   ut iaceant fusi per tua terga, veto.
Illo praecipue ne sis morosa caveto
   tempore, nec lapsas saepe resolve comas.
Tuta sit ornatrix: odi, quae sauciat ora
   unguibus et rapta bracchia figit acu. 240
Devovet, ut tangit, dominae caput illa, simulque
   plorat in invisas sanguinolenta comas.
Quae male crinita est, custodem in limine ponat
   orneturue Bonae semper in aede Deae.
Dictus eram subito cuidam venisse puellae: 245
   turbida perversas induit illa comas.
Hostibus eveniat tam foedi causa pudoris
   inque nurus Parthas dedecus illud eat!
Turpe pecus mutilum, turpis sine gramine campus
   et sine fronde frutex et sine crine caput. 250

# Translation

I begin with cultivation: from grapes well cultivated Liber
   gives good vintage, and on cultivated ground the crop stands high.
Beauty is a divine gift; how few girls can pride themselves on beauty?
   A great part of you all lack such a gift.

Care will bestow beauty; beauty neglected will go to waste, 105
    though it even be that of the Idalian goddess.
If girls of old did not cultivate their bodies thus,
    the girls of old did not have men cultivated thus.
If Andromache were dressed in a stout tunic,
    why be amazed? She was the wife of a tough soldier. 110
No doubt, as his wife you would have come dressed up to Ajax,
    he for whom seven hides of oxen were a covering!
There was raw plainness before; now Rome is golden
    and possesses the great wealth of the conquered world.
Look now at what the Capitol is, and what it was: 115
    you would say they belonged to different Jupiters.
The Curia is now most worthy of so great a council,
    when Tatius held the kingship it was made from straw.
The Palatine that now gleams under Phoebus and our leaders,
    what was it but a pasture for oxen intended for ploughs? 120
Let ancient times please others, I rejoice that I was not born until
    now: this age is suited to my ways,
not because now pliant gold is dragged from the earth
    and a pearl comes gathered from an alien shore,
not because mountains shrink as the marble is dug out, 125
    not because cerulean waters are dispersed by masonry,
but because cultivation is here and rusticity
    has not remained into our days, surviving our grandfathers.

You too must not weigh down your ears with expensive gems,
    which the discoloured Indian gathers in green water, 130
and do not go forth laden with garments embroidered in gold:
    the wealth, through which you seek us, often repels.
We are captured by simple elegance: let your locks not be without rule;
    the application of hands can give and also deny beauty.
Nor is there but one form of adornment: let each girl choose 135
    what is becoming to her and take counsel before her own mirror.
An oval face commends the parting of an unadorned head:
    Laodamia had locks arranged thus.

A small knot to be left for them at the top of the forehead,
   so that the ears might show forth, round faces desire.    140
Let one girl's hair hang down over either shoulder:
   thus are you, melodious Phoebus, when you have taken up the lyre.
Let another girl have her hair tied back in the fashion of girt Diana,
   as she is accustomed, when she hunts frightened beasts.
For this one it is becoming to let her flowing locks lie loosely,    145
   let that one be restrained with tresses tightly bound.
It pleases this one to be adorned by a Cyllenaean tortoise shell,
   let that one support folds similar to waves.
But as you will never count the acorns on the branchy oak,
   nor how many bees are in Hybla nor how many beasts in the Alps,    150
neither is it possible for me to count so many styles by number:
   every next day adds fashions.
Even neglected hair becomes many: often you would believe
   it lay loose from yesterday, it just recently having been combed afresh.
Let art imitate chance: when Alcides saw Iolé thus    155
   after capturing her city, he said, 'I love this girl'.
In such a guise, abandoned girl of Cnossos, did Bacchus
   lift you into his chariot, with Satyrs shouting '*euhoe*'.
O, how much does nature indulge your charm,
   whose losses can be atoned for in multiple ways!    160
We are shamefully laid bare, our hairs carried away by time,
   keep falling, as when Boreas shakes off the leaves.
A woman dyes the grey with German herbs,
   and by means of art achieves a better colour than the true one;
a woman goes out covered entirely with purchased locks and    165
   instead of her own, with money, she makes the locks of others her own.
Nor is there blushing at having bought them: we see them purchased openly
   before the eyes of Hercules and the Virgin band.

What shall I say about clothes? Not you, brocades, do I need
   nor you, wool, blushing with Tyrian dye.    170
Since so many colours have come out at a cheaper price,

what madness is it to carry one's entire wealth on the body?
Behold the colour of the sky at the time when the sky is without clouds
   and the warm south wind is not beckoning rainy showers;
behold the colour similar to you, who are said to have once snatched     175
   Phrixus and Helle from the snares of Ino.
This colour imitates the waves, and takes its name too from the waves:
   I could believe the Nymphs to be covered by this raiment;
that one is similar to saffron (in a saffron-hued shawl is veiled
   the dewy goddess when she yokes the light-bringing horses),     180
this one to Paphian myrtles, this one to purple-hued amethysts
   or white roses or the Thracian crane.
Nor, Amaryllis, are your chestnuts lacking, nor almonds,
   and wax has given its own name to fleeces.
As many as the blossoms the new earth produces, when in warm spring     185
   the vine stirs its buds and sluggish winter has fled,
as many and more juices the wool drinks up: choose individual ones,
   for not every colour will be suited to every girl.
Dusky tones flatter snow-white girls: dusky tones were flattering on Briseis;
   when she was carried off, she was in a dusky robe.     190
Whites flatter dark girls: in white, daughter of Cepheis, you were pleasing;
   clothed thus by you was Seriphos trodden.

How close I came to warning you, no fierce goat should make its way under
   the arms nor should your legs prickle with coarse hair!
But I am not instructing girls from the Caucasian cliffs,     195
   nor the likes of those who drink your waters, Mysian Caicus.
Why should I teach that laziness should not darken the teeth,
   and that the face should be washed with water taken up in the morning?
You also know how to obtain dazzling whiteness from applying chalk;
   she who does not blush from true blood, blushes by means of art.     200
By means of art you fill up the bare boundaries of the eyebrow
   and a small patch covers cheeks to make them look unblemished.
Nor are you ashamed to accentuate the eyes with delicate ash
   or with saffron born near you, shining Cydnus.

There is a little book of mine, in which I spoke of treatments for 205
   your looks, small, but in regards to the care, a great work.
In there also seek assistance for damaged beauty;
   my art is not idle when it concerns your interests.
Nevertheless a lover should not catch the boxes exposed on
   the table: the concealment of art aids your appearance. 210
Who would not be offended by muck smeared all over the face,
   when having slipped because of its weight, drips onto a warm bosom?
How the wool-grease stinks, though the oil extracted from
   the sheep's unwashed fleece be sent from Athens!
I would not approve of blended hind marrow being applied in front 215
   of others nor teeth cleaned in front of others.
Such things will bestow beauty, but will be unbeautiful to the sight,
   and many things, while foul when being done, are pleasing when done.
The statues of industrious Myron that now are famous,
   were once a lifeless lump and a hard mass. 220
Gold is first beaten, so that it may become a ring;
   the garments that you wear, were once dirty wool.
The stone was rough, while being made; now it is a noble signet-ring,
   with a naked Venus wringing out the sea-water from her moist locks.
While you also are in the process of cultivation, let us think you are 225
   asleep: more appropriately will you be perceived after the final touch
   of the hand.
Why must the cause of the whiteness in your face be known to me?
   Close the door of the bedroom: why do you show the unfinished product?
It is proper that men remain ignorant of many things; the greatest part of
   things would offend, if you do not conceal your secrets in your
   chamber. 230
If you examine the golden statues that shine in the decorated theatre,
   you will despise them: gold-leaf conceals the wood.
But it is not permitted for people to go near them, unless they are
   completed, nor must beauty be contrived unless men are kept away.

But I forbid you *not* to offer your locks to be combed in public, 235
   so that they hang rippling over your shoulders.

Beware especially lest being bad tempered
  at that time, and do not continually undo any escaped locks.
Let the hairdresser be unharmed: I hate the girl who wounds faces
  with nails and with a snatched hairpin stabs arms.                    240
As she touches the head of her mistress she curses it, and at the same time
  blood-stained, she weeps over the hated locks.
Let her whose hair is insufficiently thick, place a guard at the door
  or always be coiffured in the temple Bona Dea.
My arrival was suddenly announced once to a certain girl:              245
  in her confusion she threw on her locks all askew.
Let such a cause of a foul shame befall my enemies
  and let that disgrace pass to the young girls of Parthia!
Ugly is a hornless ox, ugly is a field without grass
  and a plant without leaves and a head without hair.                  250

## Commentary

In *Amores* 1.14, Ovid's position on cosmetics is carefully nuanced; substances need to be applied that will enhance naturally beautiful features, to wit, Corinna's hair, and over application or ill-advised choices can end in disaster. The advice: careful planning and, above all, an awareness of the refinements of *cultus*. The same message is conveyed in the last Book of the *Ars*. Dedicated to female readers, expressly *libertinae*, including *meretrices* (cf. above pp. 20–21), Book Three is an extensive and exhaustive series of advice, characterized by erotically-charged intent. In keeping with the generic qualities of didactic and erotodidactic poetry, the three books of the *Ars* provide a catalogue-style approach to their subject matter, with long lists of thematic advice interspersed with *exempla*, often of a mythic and legendary nature, which is suitably Alexandrian. This approach is also a feature of the *Medicamina* and the *Remedia*, as is the proliferation of a technical vocabulary (less so in the *Remedia*), which not only acknowledges the genre but also showcases knowledge (cf. Gibson 2003: 11–13).

This selection from *Ars* Book Three, *ll*.101–250, belongs to part one of Ovid's instructions, which deals with the theme of *cultus*. It is introduced at *ll*.99–100, and concludes at *l*.380. It is followed by a transitional passage, *ll*.381–498, which leads to part two, *ll*.501–808, also marked by an introduction at *ll*.499–500. Part two of the advice covers what Gibson defines as 'advanced instruction' (Gibson 2003: 2), Ovid's *maiora* ('greater things', *l*.499). These involve advice on making the most of each sexual partner, the best ways to treat younger and older lovers, dealing with rivals as well as bedroom techniques. The essence of the structure points to the necessity of acquiring *cultus* before the hunt for an *amator* can begin.

## Lines 101–106 – In praise of cultivation and beauty

*cultus* is listed as an important weapon for women to conquer men, hence Ovid's authoritative statement: *ordior a cultu* ('I begin with cultivation'). The section that follows is lengthy and varied, including advice on hair, clothing, hygiene and facial beautification (*ll*.133–250). It is extended at *ll*.251–380 to provide tips on posture, voice and other matters of *cultus*.

In *Med. ll*.3–24, Ovid writes of the cultivation of the land, the advancements in architecture and transformation of natural objects, the age of Tatius and early rusticity, and then the cultivated girls of his own era. Similarly, in *AA* 3.101–120 he writes about the land, women and cultivation, and then turns his attention to the past. Both passages illustrate the evolutionary process of *cultus* and establish a thematically effective background to the ensuing advice in each poem.

The reference to Liber (Bacchus) springing forth and providing a good grape harvest is part of Ovid's rhetorical device to set-up a convincing argument for the care of the self. As uncultivated land will result in a poor harvest and a cultivated field will flourish, beauty (*forma*, twice in *l*.103) will go to waste if neglected. Of course, not all women possess *forma* because it is a divine gift. Nevertheless, all women want beauty. The advice, therefore, caters mainly to those not blessed with beauty; but even those few who are natural beauties will benefit from heeding his instructions.

## Lines 107–128 – The past and the present

Like the Sabine matron and her daughter in *Med. ll*.11–16, the girls of long ago in *AA* 3.107–108 are found wanting in *cultus*. They were indifferent to their *corpora* ('bodies') because their husbands were indifferent to *cultus*. To illustrate the point, Andromache and Tecmessa are introduced (*ll*.109–112). Andromache, in a stout tunic, complements Hector's tough character, while adornment for Tecmessa would be wasted on a man like Ajax whose preference is for rawhide. Both women are as well matched to their husbands as the elegant *puellae* of the *Medicamina* are matched to theirs. The *exempla* are part of Ovid's rejection of the past, beginning at *ll*.113–114:

> simplicitas rudis ante fuit; nunc aurea Roma est
>     et domiti magnas possidet orbis opes.

> There was a raw plainness before; now Rome is golden
>     and possesses the great wealth of the conquered world.

The contentious sentiments of these lines are conveyed by their implicit redefinition of what constitutes an ideal (and idealized) past. For the poet of the *Ars*, the past was not some pre-agricultural, pre-technological utopia or Golden Age, but a time without *cultus* and *ars* – a time of *simplicitas rudis* ('raw plainness'). As Gibson (2003: 134) notes, *ll*.113–114 are meant to be juxtaposed to corresponding passages from Virgil, Tibullus and Propertius. Virgil's description of Evander's settlement emphasizes its primitiveness in order to press the theme of the evolution of Rome from humble beginnings (*Aeneid* 8.347–348). When pointing out the original Capitol, Virgil notes that it is *aurea nunc* ('gold now'), but was once overrun with thorn bushes. Tibullus 2.5 presents an even more romantic vision of the old city at the time of Aeneas, with cattle grazing on the Palatine (*l*.25) and scattered huts on the Capitol (*l*.26). After a series of images of bucolic peace, he sings of the city that will rise and rule the world (*ll*.56–57). Propertius dedicates several poems to the same theme in Book 4 (4.1, 4.2, 4.4 and 4.9).

In contrast, Ovid's comparisons between old and new Rome, heralded at *ll*.113–114, and continued in *ll*.115–120, extol the new city – not by an exclusive focus on its near miraculous growth from a rough but admirable culture – but by an exuberant dismissal of the primitivism of the olden days. The Curia, now the site of great debates, was made of straw in the age of Tatius. The Palatine, now housing the gleaming Temple of Apollo, once pastured oxen (the couplet, cast as a rhetorical question, underscores the unimpressive rusticity of the site's shabby history).

At *ll*.121–122, Ovid claims that idealizing times past are for those poetic predecessors from whom he departs; he enjoys living *nunc* ('now') because it is suited to his *mores* ('ways'). Somewhat surprisingly, he then turns his attention to the unnatural processes behind the technological advancements of modern Rome, with an emphasis on the means by which luxury items such as gold, pearls and marble are obtained (*ll*.123–126). This may seem puzzling in view of his admiration for the beautification of the city, which, by necessity, has required mining, imports and quarries (*ll*.123–125). Admiration of architectural engineering but dislike of villas extending into the sea (*l*.126) may seem equally perplexing. The mystery inherent in the juxtaposition of two seemingly conflicting attitudes in *ll*.113–120 and *ll*.123–126 is aggravated by cross-referencing the latter lines with *Med. ll*.7–10 where gold mining, marble quarrying, Tyrian cloth and ivory ornamentations are endorsed as markers of cultivation.

The reason for the apparent internal contradiction in *AA* 3.113–126 is most likely rhetorical. The goal of *Ars* Book Three is to establish a persuasive, possibly definitive definition of *cultus* for the modern woman. This definition is partly comprised of what it excludes: any romantic notions about the charm of the past (*ll*.113–120) and any greedy notions about the luxury of the present (*ll*.121–126). Afterwards, Ovid can proceed to detailed instruction.

Regarding the contrast between *AA* 3.121–126 and *Med. ll*.7–10, as the goals of the *Medicamina* are to instruct women in the pleasures of *cultus* and to encourage them to try his recipes, Ovid needs persuasive rhetoric, and *ll*.7–10 may be nothing more. Additionally, some four years have passed between the two works, marking a development in Ovid's definition of *cultus*.

On the scholarly discussions of these passages, cf. Watson (1982); Nikolaidis (1994); Gibson (2003: 144–145).

## Lines 129–134 – Don't over-accessorize

The advice to women begins with what *not* to wear, namely luxurious jewellery (heavy gem earrings) and clothing (gold-embroidered garments). In view of the previous discussion of *ll*.121–126, this is not surprising.

In the second half of *l*.133 Ovid advises that women's *capilli* should not be unrestrained or without *lex* (lit. 'law', here translated as 'rule') if their goal is to attract men. Following on, at *l*.134 he proffers the maxim: *admotae formam dantque negantque manus* ('the application of hands can give and also deny beauty'). These two references to hair mark the transition to *ll*.135–168 on Ovidian *coiffure des arts*.

## Lines 135–168 – Hair

The advice is to examine oneself in a mirror to see which hairstyle will suit's one's features. Ovid provides advice on styles that compliment two different facial shapes, oval and round, then lists examples of various types of coiffure, incorporating examples of certain heroines and deities for illustration. Interspersed are references to the plethora of styles and men's struggle with baldness (prompting a discussion of dyes and wigs):

(i) An oval face. To avoid accentuating an oval face, a woman should favour a parting of the hair in the middle of an unadorned head. Ovid uses the noun *discrimen* ('that which parts') to note the use of a comb or hair pin. Gibson (2003: 151) suggests that the noun also implies Ovid's familiarity with the hair ornament, the *discriminale*. On the latter, Isidorus (*Etymologiae* 19.31) writes:

> Discriminalia capitis mulierum sunt vocata ex eo, quod caput auro discernant, nam discriminare dividere dicitur.
> 
> 'Discriminalia' of women's heads are so-called because they divide the head with gold, for 'discriminare' means 'to divide.'

While Isidorus describes the *discriminale* as golden, this type of jewellery could include precious stones (as per Gibson 2003: 151 with references). Gibson argues that Ovid includes the secondary reference to the *discriminale* with a tone of disapproval because the accessory equates to luxury. This is borne out by the adjective *purum* ('unadorned') to describe the *caput* ('head') and the example of the heroic archetype – Laodamia – newly-wed wife of Protesilaus. She parted her hair thus and clearly saw no need to accentuate her style with a piece of fancy jewellery. That Ovid clearly regarded her as an austere, modest figure is attested by his earlier portrayal of her at *AA* 3.17–18 as well as in *Her.* 13, particularly *ll*.31–32 where she refuses to have her hair styled or to wear golden clothes.

(ii) A round face. This facial shape is best suited to the *nodus* ('frontal knot') style in which a section of hair was rolled over the forehead to form a toupee, then drawn back to join the rest of the hair in a bun (Leary 1990: 153). The roll of hair, pulled back from the face would lengthen its shape by accentuating the forehead, while the styling of the hair into a bun, which exposes the ears, would add additional proportion. The *nodus* was made popular by Augustus's wife, Livia, and his sister, Octavia, and numerous busts depict them with this style.

(iii) Over the shoulder. A style that was popular in statuary depictions of various gods, including Apollo. The Kassel Apollo, a series of replicas of a Greek original by Pheidias, depicts the god with long curls placed behind the ears and locks over each shoulder. Wood (2000: 229) suggests that this style, based on such statuary, may well have been the source of inspiration for the hair of Agrippina the Elder (as depicted in various busts).

(iv) Tied back. Apollo's sister, Diana, is the inspiration for this simple, practical bun.

(v) Free. In contrast to the 'Diana' style is the neglected, uncombed look (cf. *Am.* 1.14.19–20). While the 'look' is natural, the hair has been styled. *cultus* in this respect can be deceptive; contrivance is needed to look uncontrived.

(vi) Constricted. Essentially repeating Diana's style with one subtle distinction: in the Diana imagery, the hair is tied back, 'out of the way' (Gibson 2003: 154) as indicated by the verb *religare*, while here the hair is restricted by means of binding, indicated by *impedire*. The implication is that the hair itself is used to achieve the constricted style.

(vii) Ornamented. Mercury, born on Mt Cyllene in Arcadia, created the lyre from a tortoise shell; hence the adjective 'Cyllenaean' for a hair ornament. Like ivory (*Med. l.*10), tortoise shell was widely used for ornamentations for an elite market.

(viii) Curls. As *sinus* can designate something that is rounded, folded or hollowed, here it designates curled or coiled hair. Prepared in tight curls, the hair can then be pinned to achieve a 'wave' effect. This style may foreshadow the more extravagant coiffures of the later imperial period such as the one preferred by Julia Domna that was achieved by wearing a globular-shaped, towering wig fashioned from numerous tight curls (cf. the Fonseca Bust). The curling iron, required for such a style, is discussed on pp. 93–94; cf. also Fig. 6 (the *calamistrum* is to the right of the mirror, under the comb).

As waves are never-ending, so too are women's hairstyles and at *ll.*149–152 Ovid takes a detour to discuss the multiplicity of options. There are as many styles as there are acorns on the oak, bees in Sicilian Hybla and beasts in the Alps. For points of imitation, cf. Gibson (2003: 155–156). As in *Am.* 1.14.41 with its verbal amulet – *procul omen abesto* ('let such an ill be far away') – here Ovid employs the caveat, *nec ... fas est* ('nor is it wise'), which is aligned with traditional religion rather than magic. As Catullus employs the phrase in almost identical form at 51.2 in an effort to avoid punishment for comparing a man to the gods, Ovid acknowledges (humorously) that calculating the number of hairstyles is as unwise or conceited an act, and thus potentially as punishable, as challenging divine precepts. Gibson (2003: 156) explains that the phrase 'is conventionally used in the context of revealing the mysteries'.

(ix) Neglected. Similar to the free style of *l.*145. *neglecta* signals indifference but the reference to the hair having been recently combed back (*repectere*) again accentuates the deception inherent in *cultus*. According to Ovid at *l.*155, *ars* should imitate *casus* ('chance'). The maxim is introduced to reinforce his views on this style and two mythological *exempla* are cited: Iolé and Ariadne. Alcides (Hercules' original name) saw Iolé with *genuinely* neglected hair because of the sack of her home, Oechalia, and was immediately smitten, exclaiming *amo* ('I am in love'); cf. Gibson (2003: 157) on Ovid's alteration of the myth to suit his argument. Similarly, Bacchus, upon seeing Ariadne with neglected hair after Theseus abandoned her, claims her immediately. Ovid's penchant for the sensuality of vulnerable, abandoned and dishevelled women is perhaps best demonstrated in his retelling of the rape of the Sabine women at *AA* 1.101–134; cf. also *Am.*1.8 and 2.4.

At *ll.*159–168 Ovid concludes this section with the second digression, namely that women, unlike men, can do something about loss or greyness of hair. This leads back to more (indirect) advice on women's hair, namely dyes and wigs that were 'part of the package of cosmetic *colores* identified and satirised in love elegy' (Bradley 2009: 176).

Ovid delivers *ll.*159–160 in a quasi-religious tone. *natura* ('nature') – a personified or sentient force here – gives women the gift of *decus* ('charm') and if that gift is not complete, if *damna* ('losses') are present, women must atone for them. The witty implication is that recourse to *cultus* in the form of hair dyes and wigs constitutes propitiation not vanity. The rhetorical nature of Ovid's approach to this didactic philosophy is exhibited in the case study of men: nature does not favour their beauty as much because they go bald (*ll.*161–162). While Ovid suggests that men do not have access to such means of propitiation, this is untrue (as Ovid was well aware); some men did dye their hair, others wore wigs, and there are numerous recipes for curing baldness in medical and related texts. On cures for alopecia, cf. for example, Galen (12.403–404 Kühn 1826) on a recipe by Cleopatra that involved powdered realgar (or ruby sulphur) and oak coppice applied to a scalp that had been washed with soda (Galen added natron to the mix, claiming it worked well). A more exotic recipe listed by Galen (12.404 Kühn 1826) included burnt mice and wine dregs among other things. Of course, men who dyed their hair or applied unguents to conceal baldness were regularly a source of ridicule; cf., for example, Martial 6.57 and 6.74.

Wigs are another option available to women to atone for any hair defects. Ovid also emphasizes that there should not be any embarrassment about purchasing wigs because women openly visit their purveyors near the temple of Hercules and the Muses in the Campus Flaminius (contra Martial 12.23). Gibson (2003: 161) suggests that the shops 'were perhaps located in the *porticus Philippi* built around the temple.' Further on hair dye and wigs, cf. pp. 87–88 and pp. 95–96. For a contra view to Ovid's endorsement, cf. above pp. 7–8; Martial 12.23.1.

## Lines 169–192 – Clothes and colours

What shall Ovid say about clothes? Quite a lot as it transpires. His message, however, is elementary and comes in the form of Ovid's version of the modern-day colour-wheel used by stylists to ensure women's clothes match their complexions.

Harlow (2012: 42) and Bradley (2009: 179) discuss the imitation of Plautus's *Epidicus ll.*223–234. While the list of fabric colours in the play is designed as a comic attack on women's fashions, Ovid's list is not. This contrast in attitude may well be why Ovid chose such an overt example of imitation; quite possibly prompting his readership to note the divergence from the Plautine text, which seems somewhat old fashioned and tired in the context of Ovid's fresh approach to the subject.

As in *ll*.129–132, this new section begins with what to avoid. Clothing trimmed with *segmenta* (translated here as 'brocades'; strips of fabric, ornamentations on the hems of clothing) and dyed with costly *murex* are unnecessary. Not only are they ostentatious, but cheaper imitations of such expensive colours are available. On gold dresses and red dye from *murex*, cf. p. 51 and p. 49, respectively. On dyed wool, cf. Sebesta (1994: 66) who comments that 'the Romans preferred to dye the fleece rather than the cloth', further noting that available dyes worked well with wool in comparison to materials such as linen. The colouring of the wool with *murex* makes it blush (*rubere*) at *l*.170.

After this, the multiplicity of colours and shades begins at *l*.173. Ovid does not specify colour terms but employs nature-based and myth-based similes to suggest the beauty of the colours, shades and hues of fabrics. This approach to communicating colour recalls the similes used to describe Corinna's hair at *Am*. 1.14.9–12; the uniqueness of each dyed cloth, like the uniqueness of the colour of the hair, ultimately defies the employment of pedestrian colour terminologies:

(i) The colour of *aer* / 'the sky' (*ll*.173–174). Ovid uses the adjective *aerius* ('pertaining to the sky or the air'), which 'is not actually attested in references to a sky-blue colour' but 'may have been current in technical language.' (Gibson 2003: 165). Sebesta (1994: 68) suggests the colour is light-blue.

(ii) The colour of Nubes (*ll*.175–176). The cloud goddess, Nubes or Nephele, rescued her children, Phrixus and Helle from the snares of their wicked stepmother, Ino, by sending a flying golden ram to carry them to safety (later dedicated to Aeëtes as the Golden Fleece). As it is impossible, without recourse to poetic imagery, to evoke the colour of the sky on a cloudless day, it is equally impossible to adequately describe the tone of clouds. Quite likely, the tone suggested here is akin to grey.

(iii) The colour of *undae* / 'waves' (*ll*.177–178). A reader may ask: 'what is the colour of waves?' Ovid may answer 'the colour worn by sea nymphs' (*l*.178) because he is 'evoking a much broader visual paradigm than "sea-blue (green)" shade' (Bradley 2009: 184). In other words, the palette range of the waves defies the exactitude of language. While possibly the reference is to sea-green or sea-blue, it is more than that – it is the freshness, the lightness of the sea-blue waves with their whitish tips.

(iv) Similar to saffron (*ll.*179–180). As this genus comes in a variety of colours, the hint that a yellow hue is being referenced is the simile of Aurora, goddess of the dawn. Scarborough (1996: 50) mentions that saffron was '*very costly*'; obtained from the 'styles of the flowers of *Crocus sativus* … it takes over 100,000 flowers to produce 1 kilogram.'

(v) The colour of Paphian myrtles (*l.*181). The reference is to the myrtles growing near the temple of Venus in Paphos (south-west of Cyprus). The dye derived from the berries is a dark green colour; Ovid refers to the myrtle as *viridis* ('green') at *Fast*. 4.139 and as *nigra* ('black') at *AA* 3.690.

(vi) The purpled-colour of amethysts (*l.*181). The phrase *purpureae amethysti* ('purple-coloured amethysts') alludes to 'a dye that evoked and counterfeited two prodigiously expensive luxuries at the same time' (Bradley: 2009: 184–185), namely the purple produced from *murex* and the expensive gem, the amethyst. On fake purple, cf. Pliny 22.3–4 who explains that a cheaper version is sourced from a crop, although people complain that the dye fades with washing. Interestingly, in the same section, Pliny observes that growing such a crop is a much safer way to access the dye as no one risks their life harvesting *murex* for a woman keen to impress her lover or for a man to ensnare another's wife.

(vii) The shade of white roses (*l.*182); not pure white (cf. Sebesta 1994: 68).

(viii) The shade of the Thracian crane (*l.*182). This shade suggests a darker grey than the whitish grey of roses.

(ix) The colour of the chestnuts (of Amaryllis) and almonds (*l.*183). A reference to the shepherdess who loved chestnuts and quinces (*Eclogues* 2.51–52). Ovid replaces the golden-yellow of a ripe quince with the creamy-brown of almonds to contrast with the rich brown of chestnuts.

(x) The colour of wax; a creamy-yellow (*l.*184).

At *ll.*185–187 the sheer multiplicity of colours begin to overwhelm Ovid and he concludes his list by exclaiming that the number equates to that of spring blossoms. The earth is presented as independently producing colourful blossoms for humans to cultivate (cf. Bradley 2009: 185 who describes the image as one of 'natural phenomenon').

Ovid advises women to be restrained when it comes to the cornucopia of available colours. Certain colours suit certain complexions and some colours are unflattering (*ll.*187–188). Two heroic examples are then furnished at *ll.*189–192: 'snow-white' (*nivea*) Briseis suited 'dusky' (*pulla*) tones, while 'dark' (*fusca*) Andromeda, daughter of Cepheus, looked good in 'white' (*alba*). Part of the Alexandrian light-heartedness of the two couplets comes from Ovid's focus on suitable colours while describing dramatic moments in the heroines' narratives. Accordingly, Briseis is colour-coordinated albeit in the process of being snatched by Achilles while Andromeda, off-set in white, looks pleasing even while scrambling over the island of Seriphos with Perseus. On the literary traditions concerning these heroines and their physical descriptions, cf. Gibson (2003: 171); on Andromeda and Perseus, cf. Ovid's *Met.* 5.236–249; on Briseis and Achilles, cf. *Her.* 3.

## Lines 193–198 – Some advice on hygiene

Not one to be daunted by sensitive topics like body odour and bad teeth, Ovid tackles them with clever posturing. He is not, after all, writing for *puellae* from Caucasus, a region between the Black and Caspian seas renowned for its formidable mountains and wild inhabitants. Nor is he writing for girls from Mysia, those from the region north-west of Anatolia. Thus, pretending to have *almost* advised about hygiene, then remembering the genteel readers of elegy, Ovid checks himself but only to proceed with the 'unnecessary' advice all the same:

(i) Body odour, expressly, underarm odour (*l.*193). Ovid compares offensive underarm odour to the stench of a goat; cf. Catullus 69.5 and Horace *Epode* 12.5 (cf. Watson 2003: 398). The goat is often used as an example of bad smells in antiquity; for example, Theophrastus (*On Odors* 13) describes the goat as having a particularly strong smell, especially when it is on heat or in poor condition. For deodorants; cf. Pliny 21.142 on applying red iris to the underarms and also chewing the plant to alleviate bad breath, and 35.185 on liquid alum for relieving perspiration and underarm odour.

(ii) Hairy legs (*l.*194). Ovid is an avid admirer of luxurious hair – on a woman's head. As for the rest of the body, here expressly the legs, he prefers hairlessness. This is in keeping with Roman (and Greek) female beauty aesthetics that privileges the removal of body hair, including pubic hair, although depilation of the genital region was not acceptable for upright women (cf. Skinner 1982: 245). The processes of depilation (removal of hair above the skin's surface) and epilation (removal of the entire hair) included scraping, singeing and the application of ointments (depilation) as well as plucking (epilation). Pliny includes recipes for both: 28.249 (hare's blood to prevent plucked hairs from regrowing); 28.255 (the blood of a wild she-goat mixed with palm seaweed); 30.132–134 (recipes involving blood and body parts of various creatures, including bats, vipers and hedgehogs); 32.136 (similar animal-derived products). Pliny also stresses that hair removal is the preserve of women even though, unfortunately, some men practise it (14.123, 26.164 and 36.154). The latter view is also shared by Ovid at *AA* 1.505–506. Further on hair removal, cf. Martial 3.74 (ointment); 10.90 (plucking); 12.32.21–22 (resin, which he finds disgusting).

(iii) Bad teeth (*l.*197). Decayed and dirty teeth were obviously commonplace in antiquity. Leary (1996: 73–74) points out that 'the methods of cleaning them were inadequate insurance against decay (even the Emperor Augustus had bad teeth: *Suetonius* 79.2).'

In a section on remedies for tooth decay, Pliny refers to various forms of *dentrificium* ('dentifrice'). Unlike modern toothpastes and polishes, Pliny's recipes (28.178–179) involve more unusual ingredients by modern standards:

> Dentes mobiles confirmat cervini cornus cinis doloresque eorum mitigat, sive infricentur sive colluantur. Quidam efficaciorem ad omnes eosdem usus crudi cornus farinam arbitrantur. Dentifricia utroque modo fiunt. Magnum remedium est et in luporum capitis cinere. Certum est in excrementis eorum plerumque inveniri ossa; haec adalligata eundem effectum habent, item leporina coagula per aurem infusa contra dolores. Et capitis eorum cinis dentifricium est adiectoque nardo mulcet graveolentiam oris. Aliqui murinorum capitum cinerem miscuisse malunt. Reperitur in latere leporis os acui simile, hoc scarifare dentes in dolore suadent. Talus bubulus accensus eos qui labant cum dolore admotus confirmat. Eiusdem cinis cum murra dentifricium est. Ossa quoque ex ungulis suum combusta eundem usum praebent, item ossa ex acetabulis pernarum circa quae coxendices vertuntur.

Loose teeth are firmed by the ash of a stag's horn, which relieves the pain of them, whether rubbed on or used as a mouthwash. For the same purpose, some regard it as more effective to grind the unburnt horn to powder. Dentifrices are made either way. Another great remedy is the ashes of the head of wolves. It is true that bones are to be found in the excrement of many of them; these, having been bound [as an amulet], have the same effect and likewise the rennet from a hare, poured in the ear, stops the pain. Also the ash of its head is a dentifrice, and with the addition of nard, reduces the offensive smell of the mouth. Some choose to add the ash from the heads of mice. Found in the flank of the hare is a bone like a needle, which is recommended to scrape teeth in pain. The ignited pastern bone of oxen applied to those that are loose and painful strengthens them. The ash of the same with myrrh is a dentifrice. Additionally, bones from the hooves of pigs when burnt have the same effect, as do the bones from the sockets of the haunches around which moves the hip-bone.

Pliny lists other remedies that clearly blend medicinal cures, cosmetics and magic (in the form of the amulet he cites). He includes hartshorn (cf. above pp. 64–65) as beneficial to damaged teeth and also as a dentifrice. As the substance when crystallized becomes ammonium carbonate (cf. p. 65), it is an effective all-purpose cleaner as well as a time-honoured remedy for healing and whitening teeth and strengthening gums. Its alkalinity neutralizes acids in the mouth that cause tooth decay, kills germs and freshens the breath. The other references to the ash of the bones (calcined) of various animals as well as hooves would have also produced the same effects. Pliny includes a recipe made from the ash of the pastern bone of an ox mixed with myrrh. This dentifrice would certainly benefit the teeth and gums as myrrh possesses anti-inflammatory and antibacterial properties (cf. pp. 76–77); it also freshens the breath and is still used to relieve mild toothache. Elsewhere, Pliny mentions *murex* (32.82) as does Dioscorides (2.4); egg and oyster shells (29.46; 32.65); natron (31.117); pumice (36.156). He also recommends toothpicks made from the bone of a hare; on toothpicks in ancient Rome, cf. Leary (1996: 73–74). Ovid's advice on bad breath and unsightly teeth are less technical; at *AA* 3.277–278 he advises those who experience halitosis to avoid speaking on an empty stomach and to keep the mouth at a distance from a lover, while at *ll*.281–282 he suggests that those with blackened or misshapen teeth should refrain from laughing.

Treatment of the teeth and gums is discussed by other authors such as Claudius's court physician Scribonius Largus, whose prescriptions are recorded in his *Compositions of Drugs*. Scribonius dedicates several chapters to dentistry and includes a recipe for a dentifrice that he claims was favoured by Augustus's sister, Octavia (Chapter 59). The recipe consists of barley flour, vinegar, honey, salt and nard (for sweetening the breath); cf. Singer and Singer (1950). For an alternative treatment, cf. Catullus 37.20 and 39.17–21 on Egnatius who rubs his teeth and gums with urine, which is cited as a Celtiberian tradition (the ammonia contained in urine being a whitener). As Leary (1996: 73–74) has commented, the treatments were not always an insurance against decay and further to this, it should be noted that excessive use of some ingredients such as egg or oyster shells would have damaged the teeth's enamel. Further on the problems of dental decay in Rome, with a focus on *Epode* 8.3, cf. Watson (2003: 295).

(iv) Washing the face (*l*.198). Here the distinction between *munditia* and *cultus* is implicit; once the face is clean (taking *munditia* as 'hygiene' rather than 'simple elegance'), cosmeceuticals and cosmetics can be applied. Thus Ovid creates a smooth segue to the topic that follows (*ll*.199–208).

## Lines 199–208 – Cosmetics

The section on cosmetics begins with topics that may have originally been included in the *Medicamina*. At *Med. ll*.99–100 Ovid mentions a woman who smeared her cheeks with poppies, which may be a reference to rouge as opposed to another cosmeceutical, thus marking the transition from cosmeceuticals to cosmetics. However, in these lines from the *Ars*, Ovid omits cosmeceuticals and deals directly with cosmetics; directing the reader to the *Medicamina* instead (cf. *ll*.205–207), which may imply that the *Medicamina* dealt exclusively with cosmeceuticals.

Several cosmetics are listed:

(i) Foundation / *creta* (*l*.199). The application of *creta* or chalk is for a dazzling whiteness (*candor*). Similar to kaolinite, a clay mineral still used in some cosmetics and toothpastes, *creta* like *cerussa* (cf. pp. 68–69) was combined with vinegar to produce a creamy, spreadable paste. Like other ingredients discussed, chalk served a variety of purposes in antiquity besides facial beautification. From cleaning fabric, to polishing items, chalk was also used in medicines. Scarborough (1996: 43) mentions that it was ingested in large quantities as a 'beneficial' cure for poison (still practised in some cultures).

(ii) Rouge (*l.*200). On the different rouges, cf. p. 80 and on the association between blushing and *pudor*, cf. p. 96.

(iii) Eyebrow-liner (*l.*201). By means of the application of a cosmetic, here referred to as *ars*, a woman could fill the space between the eyebrows. Some Romans regarded a monobrow as attractive; cf. Petronius (*Satyricon* 126); cf. also *Satyricon* 110 on Tryphaena's maid who produces 'eyebrows' (and wigs) from her make-up box (*pyxis*), which refers to a substance to paint them on. Olson (2009: 299) cites Claudian's 'Epithalamium of Honorius and Maria', which includes praise of Maria's monobrow (*ll.*268–269); cf. Gibson (2003: 177) for additional sources. This preference for the monobrow is attested in a few works of art, such as the sarcophagus portrait of the wife of Balbinus from the third century AD (cited by Stewart 2007: 30–31) and the portrait of the baker Terentius and his wife (Pompeii, AD 55–79). Incidentally, Suetonius mentions that Augustus had a monobrow (*Augustus* 79.2).

The Romans employed several substances to darken eyebrows: (a) *stibium* (lit. 'antimony', but also used generically for kohl in the context of eye cosmetics where kohl was comprised of the sulphide of antimony), cf. Pliny (33.102–103) who describes the production of *stibium* for sale in the form of cosmetic 'cakes'; (b) *fuligo* ('soot'), cf. Juvenal (2.93) on a male who uses *fuligo*; (c) *fungus* ('lamp-black') mixed with other ingredients, including *fuligo*, cf. Pliny (28.163); (d) *favilla* ('ashes'), cf., for example, Pliny (21.123) on the ashes of rose petals; (e) sundry other ingredients including crushed flies (Pliny 30.134).

(iv) Patches / *aluta* (*l.*202). Literally meaning a piece of soft pelt, *aluta* refers to items made from leather, including purses or pouches, shoes and beauty patches. Also called a *splenium*, the patch disguised unsightly blemishes and could also, when cut into appealing shapes, add its own form of adornment. Martial refers to a woman with a crescent moon on her forehead (8.33.22) and an ex-slave with a patch that disguises his branding (2.29.9). Pliny refers to their medicinal applications at 29.126 and 30.104.

(v) Eyeliner (*ll.*203–204). The recommendation consists of *favilla* (cf. above) or saffron. The delicate ash (*l.*203) would provide a grey shade, while saffron, harvested near the Cydnus River (southern Turkey), suggests 'a "natural" coloured foundation' (Gibson 2003: 178). As saffron was expensive (cf. above p. 115), eyeliner made from charred saffron would have been a high-end cosmetic.

The primary aim of both eyeliner and eyebrow-liner was to enhance the size of the eyes, as Pliny (33.102) writes:

> Vis eius adstringere ac refrigerare, principalis autem circa oculos, namque ideo etiam plerique platyophthalmon id appellavere, quoniam in calliblepharis mulierum dilatet oculos…
>
> Antimony has astringent and cooling properties but is mainly used for eye treatments, which is why most people give it the name *platyophthalmus* [wide-eye] because it is also used in *calliblephara* [eye cosmetics] of women to enlarge the eyes…

To make effective use of these products, skill in application was important. Various implements were sold for applying make-up and as most of the products for the eyes came in powdered form, a thin stick would be moistened and then dipped into the powder. The sticks were made of various materials to cater for various customers, ranging from simple wooden and bronze applicators, to ones fashioned from precious metals, stones and horn. The applicator was sometimes inside or attached to a container, similar to modern mascara tubes.

## Lines 209–234 – Conceal the arts of beautification

Ovid turns his attention to the concealment of the *ars* of *cultus*. He embraces facets of the anti-cosmetic tradition, describing the abject quality of some products and evoking an unflattering portrait of a woman performing her beauty regime. While these lines do not critique cosmetic use from a moral perspective, they communicate intense repugnance at the sight of a woman attending to her own body. Ironically, Ovid's woman in the process of beautification becomes the antithesis of beauty. The only other instance of such a dramatic departure from his usual attitude to female adornment is to be found in *Rem.* 343–356 (cf. below pp. 125–129).

To reinforce the directive of *l.*209, which expressly forbids the *puella* to allow her *amator* to catch her at her toilette, Ovid creates a vivid scenario of a man entering a woman's quarters and discovering what lies within, none of which is a pretty sight. Deception at all cost is vital in the process of beautification (*l.*210).

In contrast to the luxurious creams full of sweet smelling incense and floral ingredients in the *Medicamina*, the unappealing nature of the substances of *ll.*211–216 and the unattractive look of a woman applying them are vividly evoked:

(i) Muck (*faex*). The noun *faex* designates 'the residue of various liquids and solids, most commonly the dregs of wine, and is here apparently used as a facial preparation' (Gibson 2003: 184). Olson thinks it is rouge; cf. 2009: 297n37. The direct correlation between the substance and the woman's body is developed in *l*.212 as the *faex*, weighty and globulous, moves – as if by intent – from face to bosom.

(ii) Wool-grease or lanolin (*oesypum*) is the creamy-yellow wax secreted by the sebaceous glands of wool-bearing animals, particularly sheep. The use of *oesypum* in body creams has an extensive history and is still used today as a moisturizer, softener, balm and medicinal ointment. Dioscorides (2.74) describes the manufacture of *oesypum* and its uses in the treatment of sores, softening the skin, and as an eye medication. Pliny (29.35–37) lists the multiplicity of uses for *oesypum* and, like Ovid, mentions that the most prized *oesypum* comes from Attic sheep. Pliny also describes the production of *oesypum* and specifies that a test of its purity is a strong smell of grease and resistance to melting.

A substance such as *oesypum* would have been kept in a small, utilitarian *pyxis* (Fig. 1) or in a slightly larger, decorative container (Fig. 2). Gibson (2003: 183) comments that the *pyxis* was 'not only unwelcome evidence of the application of *ars*, but a repository of revolting substances.' Richlin (1995: 191, citing Wyke) considers the physical beauty of a large *pyxis* in the form of a cosmetic box in contrast to the abject contents of the little *pyxides* inside: 'makeup boxes often were decorated with scenes of women applying makeup ... so that, pretty on the outside, they would often have contained substances arousing the uneasy horror evoked by pollutants.' An excellent example of such a make-up box is the one from Campania around the first century AD (Fig. 3). This *pyxis* (height: 14.5 centimetres, width: 30.2 centimetres, depth: 24 centimetres), made of wood, bone and bronze, is decidedly feminine with its feet in the shape of Sirens, its front panels in the form of caryatids and the side panels (not shown) adorned with cupids. Inside is a bronze mirror, a gold ring, two silver *fibulae* covered in gold-leaf, a bone comb, a large pin, a needle, a spatula, a spindle and a small *pyxis*. Besides being a remarkable archaeological piece, the box is symbolic of a woman's interior, private life; a miniature of her personal chamber, if you will. In this sense, to open the lid of such a box and to delve into its contents is the metaphorical equivalent of a man entering a woman's boudoir and observing her in the act of devious and ugly beautification. Ovid implicitly evokes such an interpretation at *ll*.209–210.

(iii) Hind marrow (*cervae medulla*). This was widely employed in medicines and cosmetics. Dioscorides (2.77) states that hind marrow is the best quality marrow and is excellent for filling up wounds. As a beauty product / medicant, Pliny (28.185) mentions it mixed with veal suet and whitethorn leaf to heal facial problems such as sores; cf. also 28.241 (for sores in general). While many of the animal-based products employed by the ancients are far from politically correct ingredients from the perspective of modern cosmetics and topical medicants, hind tallow is still used in some athletic salves.

(iv) Cleaning teeth (*l*.216). Ovid does not discuss ingredients in this instance but rather lists teeth cleaning as something to be avoided in the presence of a lover. On ancient toothpastes and dental hygiene, cf. pp. 117–119.

Ovid reiterates his caution about revealing the secrets of the boudoir with two maxims (*ll*.217–218) followed by four rhetorical examples (*ll*.219–224). Playing with words at *l*.217, he states that what gives *forma* ('beauty') involves a process that is *deformia* ('unbeautiful') to the male gaze. Secondly, at *l*.218 he repeats his philosophy: many things are *turpia* ('foul') when being done, but give pleasure (*placere*) when completed. In short: hide the process and display the results. Not quite finished in labouring the point, he furnishes the example of the Greek sculptor, Myron (*fl*. 480–440 BC), whose works were originally lifeless masses and hard lumps of stone (*ll*.219–220). Likewise, beaten gold becomes a ring, sordid wool becomes a garment and an uncut stone becomes a gem engraved with the Venus Anadyomene motif (cf. p. 94).

Woman as an artefact – an adornment like a beautiful sculpture, a glittering ring, a lovely robe or an erotically-charged jewel – is a regular metaphor in ancient literature. The epitome of this concept is the myth of Pygmalion, chronicled in *Met*. 10.243–297, in which is recorded the memorable line: *ars adeo latet arte sua* ('thus art hides by means of its own artifice,' *l*.252), the very message of *AA* 3.209–250. Pygmalion, disenchanted with women, makes his own by making art. Ovid, keen commentator on women's physical flaws, makes his own by making manuals. Art therefore makes women and, by extension, Ovid's women by means of art make themselves.

The same theme is continued at *ll*.225–234. Interestingly, at *ll*.229–230 Ovid states that it is proper that men remain ignorant of such things – indeed, knowing about them would be a cause of offence (the *praeceptor* being an exception, obviously). Thus, to avoid giving offence, a woman must regard herself as akin to the much admired statues in theatres. The statues are made of wood but covered in gold-leaf. As people are not permitted to venture near them while they are being constructed, they remain ignorant of the wood underneath the gold. The final product of the artist, therefore, is not deemed worthless if what lies under the façade, like the creative process itself, is never seen.

## Lines 235–250 – Hairdressing

The dressing of one's hair *must* be done in the presence of the lover. But in order for the adornment to be all that it should be for the male, there are stipulations. While it is wonderful to watch a woman combing her hair and arranging it over her shoulders, she should avoid doing this when she is ill-tempered or when she is having a bad hair day. The unfortunate fate of the hairdresser who is the object of her mistress's tantrums is a motif explored elsewhere by Ovid (*Am.* 1.14) and other poets; cf. above p. 92. Ovid expands the motif by humorously suggesting that a *puella* with insufficiently thick hair, should place a guard at the door to keep out her lover, or consider being coiffured at the temple of Bona Dea on the Aventine (*l*.244), where men are forbidden. Concluding the section on hair, Ovid indulges himself with a personal anecdote; once he arrived at the door of an unnamed women and in her confusion she ruined her appearance by throwing on her hair piece awry. In Ovid's opinion, only one's enemies or the (youthful) girls of Parthia deserve such a disaster of *cultus* (*ll*.247–248). The Parthians, traditional enemies of Rome, are an appropriate simile here, particularly, as Gibson (2003: 195) notes: 'The image of Parthian women wearing wigs is perhaps a nicely pointed retaliation to Parthian claims to be shocked by Roman decadence.'

Another maxim ends the section on hair as Ovid returns to the topic of *cultus* as an improvement on nature (*ll*.249–250). His enthusiastic and powerful validation of *cultus* is evident in these lines, particularly through the repetition of *turpis* ('ugly') in *l*.249.

# 4

## *Remedia Amoris* 343–356

### Latin text

Auferimur cultu; gemmis auroque teguntur
  omnia; pars minima est ipsa puella sui.
Saepe ubi sit, quod ames, inter tam multa requiras; 345
  decipit hac oculos aegide dives Amor.
Improvisus ades, deprendes tutus inermem:
  infelix vitiis excidet illa suis.
Non tamen huic nimium praecepto credere tutum est:
  fallit enim multos forma sine arte decens. 350
Tum quoque, compositis cum collinet ora venenis,
  ad dominae vultus, nec pudor obstet, eas.
Pyxidas invenies et rerum mille colores,
  et fluere in tepidos oesypa lapsa sinus.
Illa tuas redolent, Phineu, medicamina mensas: 355
  non semel hinc stomacho nausea facta meo est.

### Translation

We are carried away by cultivation; everything is covered by
  precious stones and gold; the real girl is the smallest part of herself.
Often you should enquire, 'where is it', that thing you love, amid so 345
  many things; with this shield does rich Amor deceive the eyes.
Unexpected you must arrive, safe yourself you will catch her unarmed:
  the poor girl will be felled from her own imperfections.
Although it is not safe to trust in this rule too much:
  in fact comely beauty without art trips up many men. 350

Then also, when she is smearing her face with composite concoctions,
    you should go to the face of your mistress, undaunted by a sense of shame.
You will find jars and stuff in a thousand colours,
    and wool-grease that has slipped and dripped onto a warm bosom.
Those substances, Phineus, reek of your table:                                  355
    not only once has this caused my stomach nausea.

# Commentary

The *Remedia Amoris*, Ovid's last hurrah in erotodidactic elegy, is a somewhat nasty, cynical but nevertheless witty *riposte* to the *Ars Amatoria*. Here Ovid's antagonists are ungrateful, hurtful women (the *indignae puellae* of *l*.15) and his audience lovesick, thwarted males. As he instructed men in the *artes* of the *amator* in Books One and Two of the *Ars*, he now turns his skills as *praeceptor amoris* – or doctor (cf. above p. 21) – to cure them of the women they once sought. Henderson (1979: xx–xxii) provides a detailed analysis of the structure of the poem, which is thematically framed around a variety of techniques to rid oneself of *amor*. The passage herein is but one of numerous remedies.

*Ll*.343–356 involve a clever strategy; surprising a *puella* amid the private rituals of *cultus* and *munditia* is not only an act designed to humiliate, but also one that reiterates the deceptive nature of women. Additionally, the reader of the *Medicamina* will recall Ovid's statement that very few women are born beautiful. This latter maxim, designed as a gentle prompt to women to employ the techniques required to make them beautiful, is now alluded to in order to suggest that feminine beauty is often an artifice that conceals a hideous reality.

The context of this extract is, therefore, a vital consideration when assessing Ovid's responses to *cultus* as well as cosmeceuticals and cosmetics. If one were to discuss it in isolation, it would present a decidedly distorted interpretation of the poet's attitude towards such matters. However, within the poem itself, it merely presents another avenue for curing lovesickness and as such it is not so much a diatribe against female adornment as a tainted version of *AA* 3.101–250, particularly *ll*.209–234 and 237–246. In short: watching your *puella* apply beauty lotions is not conducive to passion; do so only if you wish to end your desires.

Within this context, Ovid treats *cultus* cynically in comparison to the *Medicamina* and *AA* 3.101–208, 235–236 and 247–250. In the age of Ovid, *cultus* is everywhere and it is seductive (*Rem. ll.*343–344). Of course, such a message is employed elsewhere but in a more subtle, complex way that disassociates female adornment and love of *cultus* from the anti-cosmetic tradition and balances endorsement of beautification with recognition of male anxiety concerning cosmetic ritual. Ovid's familiarity with the anti-cosmetic tradition and its association with deception – themes implied in *AA* Book Three – is evident in the *Remedia* in relation to the *puella* so enamoured of *cultus* that it is difficult for a man to catch a glimpse of the *real* woman (*ll.*345–346).

Ovid evokes the façade of the adorned female through the military imagery of the shield or *aegis* (*l.*346). The latter references the shield of Jupiter (*Aeneid* 8.354) and that of Minerva, with Medusa's head (*Aeneid* 8.435; *Met.* 2.754–755 and 6.78–79). From the sublime to the ridiculous, Ovid equates the powerful, authoritative *aegis* of the gods with the glittering jewellery of the *puella*. Similarly, like the soldier who arrives suddenly on the enemy, the lover must be *improvisus* ('unexpected'); on the military connotations of the adjective, cf. Henderson (1979: 85). If the lover proves to be sufficiently stealthy, he will catch the girl when she is defenceless; cf. *deprehendere* ('to catch') and *inermis* ('unarmed'). On being besieged, the unlucky girl will be 'felled' (*excidere*), which continues the martial motif. This representation of a hypothetical situation is typical of the Ovidian motif of the lover-as-soldier that characterizes, in particular, the *Amores* and the *Ars*; cf. Murgatroyd (1975); Drinkwater (2013).

The girl is 'felled' on being surprised during her toilette because her *vitia* ('imperfections') are revealed – she is devastated at being viewed in her uncultivated state. Ovid's scene at *ll.*351–357 evokes sensory images of sight, touch and smell and the *pyxides* and their revolting contents are highlighted at *ll.*353–357, matching and distorting imagery and sentiments from *AA* 3.209–234, particularly *ll.*211–212.

On this passage, Richlin (1995: 189–190) stresses the association between facial creams, poisons and magic potions, all of which are conveyed by the noun *venena*. Ovid uses the term, translated as 'concoctions', at *l.*351, thereby creating an image of the woman as seductress-poisoner-witch. The dangers implicit in the term have already been observed by Ovid in *Am*.1.14.44 where he describes Corinna's hair dye as *venena* (translated as 'poisons'); cf. above p. 95. He also employs the term at *Am*. 2.14.28 – *dira venena* ('ill-omened poisons') – to describe the mixture Corinna ingested to abort a foetus; the magical connotations are emphasized by the lines that follow, which reference Medea (as well as the story of Philomela and Procne, infamous from *Met*. 6.412–674).

In contrast to the *Medicamina*, then, the beauty products in the *Remedia* are ugly, dangerous, magical and ill-omened. This is further emphasized by the use of *medicamina* ('substances') at *Rem. l*.355 to denote something toxic, something causing a nauseating reaction, which again alludes to witchcraft, forming as it does an uneasy intertextuality with the diatribe against magic in *Med. ll*.35–42 and the dismissal of the same in *Am*. 1.4.35–44. *medicamina*, used to denote a poison and a magical substance is used at *Met*. 7.262 (on Medea) but is mostly present in post-Augustan works; cf. Valerius Flaccus 8.17 (on the *condita medicamina* or 'hidden potions' in Medea's casket); Juvenal 6.595 (on *artes* and *medicamina* to instigate an abortion); Seneca *Controversies* 7.3.4 (as a poison and aligned with *venenum*); Tacitus *Annals* 12.67 (a deadly poison).

Ovid's *puella* has been transformed into a witch or, as above, a seductress-poisoner-witch. This is in line with interpretations of the witch as a powerful embodiment of feminine abjection, the antithesis of an elite body, and one akin to what Stratton (2014: 154) describes as a form of human 'creatureliness'. The woman at her toilette, in the very act of performing erotic magic on herself by means of potions, thereby embodies the uncanny. This is suggested by the reference to the Harpies, introduced as a metaphor of repellent olfactory hyperbole.

At *ll*.355–356, Ovid equates the smell of beauty products with the table of Phineus, the blind king of Salmydessos, who was harassed by Harpies that devoured his meals, befouled the leftovers and left a stench in their wake; cf. *Met*. 7.1–4. Ovid's immediate source is Virgil's description of the Harpies as birds with maiden-like faces at *Aeneid* 3.216–218 – beings symbolic of female 'creatureliness'. The association of Harpies with 'woman-bird' also taps into the Roman belief that witches were synonymous with metamorphosis and flight. Ovid references the belief at *Am*. 1.8.13–14 when he implies that Dipsas can transform into a bird. Likewise, in an evocative scene from Apuleius's *Metamorphoses* (3.21ff.), Pamphile takes out an ointment box (*arcula*) from her *pyxides*, smears an unguent (*unguedo*) over her naked body, then transforms into an owl (*bubo*).

Brunelle (2005: 152) puts the hyperbole into a sensible context: 'Unsurprisingly, lanolin does not really smell as bad as Ovid claims: Pliny (*Nat. Hist.* 29.36) vouches for its strong odour, but to compare it to Phineus's meals, befouled by the Harpies, and to claim that one's stomach has been repeatedly upset by the smell borders on the ridiculous.' Nevertheless, the exaggeration is a symptom of Ovid's use of satire in the *Remedia*, which provides a suitable means by which his didactic doctoring can be expressed.

# 5

## *Ars Amatoria* 1.505–524

### Latin text

| | |
|---|---:|
| Sed tibi nec ferro placeat torquere capillos, | 505 |
|     nec tua mordaci pumice crura teras. | |
| Ista iube faciant, quorum Cybeleia mater | |
|     concinitur Phrygiis exululata modis. | |
| Forma viros neglecta decet; Minoida Theseus | |
|     abstulit, a nulla tempora comptus acu; | 510 |
| Hippolytum Phaedra, nec erat bene cultus, amavit; | |
|     cura deae silvis aptus Adonis erat. | |
| Munditie placeant, fuscentur corpora Campo; | |
|     sit bene conveniens et sine labe toga. | |
| †lingua ne rigeat†; careant rubigine dentes; | 515 |
|     nec vagus in laxa pes tibi pelle natet. | |
| Nec male deformet rigidos tonsura capillos: | |
|     sit coma, sit trita barba resecta manu. | |
| Et nihil emineant et sint sine sordibus ungues, | |
|     inque cava nullus stet tibi nare pilus. | 520 |
| Nec male odorati sit tristis anhelitus oris, | |
|     nec laedat naris virque paterque gregis. | |
| Cetera lascivae faciant concede puellae | |
|     et si quis male vir quaerit habere virum. | |

## Translation

But for you let there be no pleasure in curling hair with iron,     505
    nor in rubbing your legs with biting pumice.
Bid those to do so, by whom mother Cybele
    is sung with howls in Phrygian measures.
Neglected appearance becomes men; Theseus carried off
    Minos's daughter, with no hairpin to adorn his temples;     510
Phaedra loved Hippolytus, and he was not well tended by cultivation;
    Adonis born in the woods was the goddess's beloved.
Let bodies please with cleanliness, and be tanned by the Campus;
    let the toga fit well and be without stain.
Let not the tongue protrude; let the teeth be free from plaque;     515
    nor for you should a foot slide and slip about in a too roomy shoe.
Let not inflexible locks be badly mutilated by clipping:
    let the hair, let the beard be trimmed by an expert hand.
Nails should not project and should be free from dirt,
    and for you no hair should be in the nostril cavities.     520
Let not the breath of the mouth be foul and bitter of smell,
    nor the husband and the father of the flock offend the nose.
For the rest let wanton girls practise
    and whoever, scarcely a man, seeks to have a man.

## Commentary

In this advice to men, Ovid covers much terrain. Having stated his aims at *ll*.1–40, essentially how to be skilled in loving (*amandi*, *l*.1), he sets out a detailed instructive agenda ranging from places to find the right woman, various means of winning her over, emboldened physicality and, as here, correct presentation.

    Ovid's opinions on men's appropriation of *cultus* are in stark contrast to his attitude towards women and the same. Excessive *cultus* for men (or what Ovid deems to be excessive) is directly related to adornment as opposed to neatness, cleanliness and a certain ruggedness. Ovid begins this small section on the man's public body and maintenance of his private body by explicitly citing what should be avoided. Curled hair and shaved legs (*ll*.505–506) are not appropriate because they are signifiers of masculine effeminacy as symbolized in the equation of such bodies with the priests of the Phrygian goddess, Cybele (*ll*.507–508). The latter were eunuchs and as such their status in Rome was decidedly that of the 'Other', associated as they were with foreign belief systems, barbaric practices and – literally – emasculation; cf. Watson and Watson (2014:238–241). Ovid returns to the rhetorical technique of parallelism in the concluding lines of the passage, *ll*.523–524, where he cites *lascivae puellae* ('wanton girls') and male homosexuals as the rightful custodians of such forms of *cultus*.

Here, the presentation of the specific features of the processes of cultivating the body is consistent with the pieces previously discussed. For example, Ovid mentions the *calamistrum*, a topic of preoccupation at *Am*.1.14.23–30, and depilation, which he mentions in *AA*.3.194. Other features of *cultus*, and ones aligned more closely with *munditia* in the sense of hygiene, are a clean mouth (*ll*.515, 521) and a body free of bad odours (*l*.522), which are topics discussed elsewhere (oral hygiene: *AA* 3.197; also 3.277–278, 281–282; body odour: *AA* 3.193). Ovid's advice in these lines privileges male *munditia* over male *cultus*, which highlights the gender binary associated with the terms. In relation to appearance, whether it be to appeal to a woman or to conform to social expectations, a man's *munditia* is imperative. Thus, not only is Ovid instructive on olfactory matters and hygiene, he extends his advice to grooming and demeanour: hair and beard must be neatly trimmed by a proficient hand (*ll*.517–518), clothing must be well maintained and worn correctly (*ll*.514, 516), nails and nose hair must be kept under control (*ll*.519–520), the tongue should not protrude (*l*.515).

Ovid's advice for a well presented man correlates to Cicero's evocation of the ideal behaviour and self-presentation of the ideal man in *On Duties* 1.130. While this last example of *imitatio* was not included earlier in the discussion of sources for the *Remedia* – or indeed the other pieces under analysis – its novel, hybrid format, which perhaps reveals that even Cicero enjoyed Alexandrian generic experimentation, clearly appealed to Ovid. Presented as an epistle, but in essence a didactic – hence rhetorical – and philosophical document, *On Duties* is a letter to his son, Marcus, which discusses, among other topics, the concept of what is *honestas* or honourable (cf., for example, 1.4ff.). Part of Cicero's definition of the latter is the virtue of *moderatio* or moderation (cf., for example, 1.17, 24), which is a consistent theme throughout much of his writings and is, again, a topic that was to have a profound influence on Ovid's approach to *cultus, munditia* and *ars*.

Cicero (1.28) discusses the theme of *decorum* and its relation to masculine modesty (*verecundia*) in a consideration of self-presentation that is a combination of *natura* and *munditia*:

> Cum autem pulchritudinis duo genera sint, quorum in altero venustas sit, in altero dignitas, venustatem muliebrem ducere debemus, dignitatem virilem. Ergo et a forma removeatur omnis viro non dignus ornatus, et huic simile vitium in gestu motuque caveatur. Nam et palaestrici motus sunt saepe odiosiores et histrionum nonnulli gestus ineptiis non vacant, et in utroque genere quae sunt recta et simplicia laudantur. Formae autem dignitas coloris bonitate tuenda est, color exercitationibus corporis. Adhibenda praeterea munditia est non odiosa neque exquisita nimis, tantum quae fugiat agrestem et inhumanam neglegentiam. Eadem ratio est habenda vestitus, in quo, sicut in plerisque rebus, mediocritas optima est.

> Again there are two types of beauty [*pulchritudo*], of which one is charm [*venustas*], and the other is dignity [*dignitas*], we should think charm to be feminine, dignity masculine. Therefore all ornamentation that is not befitting a man should be removed from his appearance [*forma*], and he should be made wary of similar faults in gesture and movement. For the movements of the palaestra are often unpleasant and some of the gestures of actors are not free from absurdities, and in either case those things that are upright [*rectum*] and artless [*simplex*] are praised. Additionally, the dignity [*dignitas*] of one's appearance must be preserved by a wholesome complexion, a colour from the exercise of the body. To this must be added a simple elegance [*munditia*], neither obnoxious nor overly excessive, but just enough to avoid a countrified and uncivilized neglect. The same rationale is to be enacted with clothing, in which instance, as with most things, moderation [*mediocritas*] is best.

An intratextual contradiction occurs between Ovid's lines here from *Ars* Book One, with its echoes of Cicero's no-nonsense approach to male cultivation of the body, and *Med. ll*.23–26 (pp. 53–54), with the latter text presenting a more accommodating attitude than the former. A similar conundrum has been discussed earlier in relation to the internal passages of contradiction in *AA* 3 (*ll*.113–120 and *ll*.123–126) and the contradiction between *AA* 3.123–126 and

*Med. ll.*7–10. The key to understanding Ovid's different attitudes to male *cultus*, as discussed previously (pp. 17–18), is his rhetorical imperative. In the *Medicamina*, it is important for Ovid to get the girls on-board, so-to-speak, and he attempts this, in part, by stressing the need for them to match their men in beauty and elegance. Exaggeration goes a long way in Latin rhetoric, and Ovid harnesses its potential power by the remarkable evocation of the Roman dandy at *Med. ll.*25–26. *Ars Amatoria* Book One, like *Remedia Amoris*, is concerned with different – though related – matters and a different audience to the female-centred *Medicamina*. Therefore, Ovid accentuates the methodology of rhetoric by aligning it closely to declamation, to *suasoria* (a 'hortatory' or 'suasory speech'). These lines are no mere whispers in the ears of girls eager to know beauty secrets. These are the lines to be declaimed to men – as effectively communicated via the *imitatio* of Rome's most famous practitioner of hortatory speech – Cicero (cf. Labate 1984). This should come as no surprise, as Seneca the Elder (*Controversies* 2.2.12) mentions that such a style of speaking was once practised by Ovid himself.

# Appendices

## Appendix 1: Notes on the Latin texts

### *Medicamina Faciei Femineae*

**Line 25: *poliuntur*** is the reading of Heinsius adopted by Kunz (1881: 39) and Rosati (1985: 56, 66); contra Kenney (1995: 113) who reads *potientur*.

**Lines 27-28:** Kunz (1881:39), Rosati (1985: 67), García (1995: 285), Kenney (1995: 113) and Watson (2001: 464n31) draw attention to the grammatical problems of this couplet, and Kenney is right to obelize it. Some editors have also posited, on the basis of the problems, that there must be a lacuna after *l.*26, with Kunz (1881: 59-62) even suggesting that *ll.*26-27 are most likely an interpolation. Each scholar attempts to resolve the matter by punctuation that joins *refert* at *l.*28 with the hexameter of *l.*27. The lines have been left untranslated herein.

**Line 31: *quaecumque*** is read with ***voluptas***; contra *cuicumque* read with *sibi* as per Kenney (1995: 113) and Mozley-Goold (1979: 4). Both Kunz (1881: 62) and Rosati (1985: 68) accept *quaecumque* with *voluptas*, arguing that there are no major grammatical problems.

**Line 34: *muta ... avis*** is adopted by most editors (Kunz 1881, Rosati 1985, Kenney 1995); cf. also Heldmann (1982) for a detailed defence. Kunz (1881: 40) notes several manuscripts read *multa ... avis* ('many ... a bird'), which does not make sense after the specificity of *l.*33 (namely, *the* peacock).

**Line 35: *nos urget*** as per Rosati (1985: 56) and García (1995: 285). Other readings include: *nos urat* (Heinsius); *consurget* (Kunz 1881: 40); *nos uret* (Mozley 1962: 4); *iungendus* (Mozley-Goold 1979: 4); *vos urget* (Kenney 1995: 113).

**Line 51: *discite*** repeats the opening word of the poem and is found in several manuscripts listed by Kunz (1881: 42). Kunz (42), Rosati (1985: 56) and Kenney (1995: 114) read *dic age*. Rosati (1985: 72) represents *ll*.51–52 as direct speech to argue that the lines are spoken by Venus, citing *AA* 3.43 where the goddess orders the poet to give instruction; cf. Gibson (2003: 104–5) for a discussion of the passage from the *Ars*.

**Line 60:** editors raise the problem of punctuation at *l*.60. Punctuation after *contere* is required and herein a hyphen has been inserted. While Kenney (2004) is rightly concerned that the necessary punctuation causes ambiguity as to the substance to be added, *in haec* has been taken as a reference to the dry ingredients prepared in *ll*.53–58, hence the translation of the line reads: 'see that a sixth of a whole *as* [i.e. of the crushed horn] goes in [i.e. into the vetch and barley].'

**Line 65: *trahat*** indicates 'draw out' or 'weigh'; also at *l*.80 and *l*.92. Translated in these lines as 'weigh out', 'weighs' and 'weighing' respectively to emphasize that it is an action being performed.

**Line 72: *pigris*** as per Kenney (1995: 115), rather than *nigris* as per Kunz (1881: 43) and Rosati (1985: 58).

**Line 85: *radenti tubera*;** contra Kenney (1995: 115) who adopts *rodenti corpora*. *radenti corpora* is adopted by Rosati (1985: 78–9), who notes the overlap between the two verbs, but posits that *radere* is more appropriate as it suggests the process of smoothing the skin while vigorously washing it (*rodere* appears to be too harsh a process for facial beautification, lending itself more to a medical procedure).

**Line 86: *utrimque*** follows Heinsius, Kunz (1881: 45), Rosati (1985: 58) and Kenney (1995: 115). Kenney notes that the alternative, *utrumque* 'does not seem … to be possible Latin: can an ingredient 'be' a weight? Heinsius's *utrimque*, one *hasta* different, sets the matter right literally at a stroke.'

**Line 98: *nullus*** has been adopted to govern *color* as opposed to *multos*. *nullus* is adopted by Kunz (1881: 77–8), Rosati (1985: 60) and Kenney (1995: 6); contra Mozley-Goold (1979: 8). The meaning of the line varies significantly depending on what adjective is adopted: *nullus* indicates that the skin would be colour-free, meaning blemish-free, and thus ready for the application of make-up; in contrast, *multus* denotes a face full of colour, namely, a healthy glow, after the cream has been applied. As Ovid has used ingredients known for their ability to reduce spots and facial markings, *nullus* seems the appropriate choice.

### *Amores* 1.14

**Line 4:** McKeown (1989: 2: 366) draws attention to the problems of punctuation. He cites Kenney (1958: 58), who comments that 'there is much to be said for not punctuating at all in such sentences.' In his second edition of the text, Kenney (1995: 32) prints the line without punctuation, a procedure adopted here.

**Line 21:** *Thracia* is adopted now by most commentators as opposed to the variant form, *Threcia*; contra Showerman-Goold (1977: 372) who read *Threcia*. McKeown (1989: 2: 372) notes that *Thracia* is supported by the manuscripts at *Ep.* 1.4, *Met.* 6.661 and 11.92.

**Line 24:** *mala* in preference to *male* as per Kenney (1958: 58) who aligns *quanta* with *quot*. He argues that if *quanta* were taken alone, the line would have to mean *quam inmania*, 'and editors who adopt it cite no parallels'; further, cf. Kenney (2004: unpaged). Barsby (1973: 150–1) and McKeown (1989:2: 373) adopt the same reading; contra Showerman-Goold (1977: 372) who read *male*.

**Line 46:** *tuta* causes no problems (in keeping with the concept of protecting or safeguarding one's beauty). Kenney (1958: 58) rightly draws attention to *Med.* l.1–2, *AA* 3.207 and *Rem.* l.347 for the same idea.

### *Ars Amatoria* 3.101–250

**Line 155:** *casum simulet* as per Kenney (1995: 191) and Gibson (2003: 157), the jussive subjunctive ensuring a sensible segue to the examples of Hercules and Iolé (*ll*.155–156), and Bacchus and Ariadne (*ll*.157–158). Mozley-Goold (1979: 128) reads *simulat* with the accusative, which as Gibson argues, 'lacks the point'.

**Line 158:** *Cnosi* per Kenney (1995: 191) and Gibson (2003: 158). The translation references Gibson's version of the couplet.

**Line 213:** *mittatur* as per Kenney (1995: 193) is adopted rather than *mittantur*. Gibson (2003: 184) adopts the latter: *oesypa quid redolent quamvis mittantur Athenis, / demptus ab immundo vellere sucus ovis!* Gibson's edit causes a disjointed effect (and an awkward translation). However, the exclamation at the end of the pentameter, as he suggests, makes better sense than Kenney's question mark.

**Line 231: *splendent*** as per Goold (1965: 80–1) who presents a convincing case in support of Burman's (1727) reading; cf. also Gibson (2003:190). Contra *pendent* (Kenney 1995: 194).

**Line 241: *ut*** as per Heinsius; cf. Goold (1965: 81) and Gibson (2003: 194). Contra Kenney's emendation to *et*.

## Remedia Amoris 343–356

**Line 351: *cum collinet*** is metrically sound as opposed to, for example, *cum linet* from the Monacensis 14809, saec. xii manuscript (cf. Kenney 1995: 240). *sua cum linet* preserves the metre but further problematizes the line by the inclusion of the unnecessary pronoun, which is described by Henderson (1980: 162) as 'totally otiose'. Goold (1965: 99–101) argues convincingly for *cum collinet*, pointing out the contextual soundness of the verb as well as its contribution to 'the successive gutturals' of *quoque compositis cum collinet*, which he exemplifies by the translation: 'when caking her cheeks with crude concoctions.' (Ibid. 101). Kenney was not initially in support of the reading (1961: 578n1) but does adopt it in his second edition (1995: 240). Cf. also Henderson (1980: 162) in support of *collinet*.

## Ars Amatoria 1.505–524

**Line 515:** †**lingua ne rigeat**† is problematic. As Hollis (1977: 120) has discussed, it would make sense to assume the whole line refers to oral hygiene; cf., therefore, Kenney (1995: 142), where the clause is obelized and reads *lingua ne rigeat*. Contra Goold (1965: 65–6) who endorses Palmer's emendation, *lingula ne ruget* ('let not the shoe-strap be creased'), with the maintenance of the verb, *rigeat* ('let not the shoe-strap be tied too tight'). Thus, the remainder of the line – *careant rubigine dentes* – can be rendered as 'keep the teeth [of the buckle] free from stain', which then links the imagery to the pentameter of *l*.516. This latter reading seems overly forced, and accepting Kenney's reading still maintains any conscious *double entendre* of *l*.515, particularly in the context of *l*.516.

# Appendix 2: Glossary of cosmeceutical terminology

***Astringent:*** a product that shrinks or tightens body tissues and dries up secretions.

***Cleanser:*** a product made from natural and / or synthetic ingredients to clean the face and / or the body by removing dirt, dead skin cells, sweat, excess oils and bacteria. The process of cleansing unblocks pores and prevents or reduces skin conditions such as acne. Cleansers are removed with water.

***Decoction:*** a method of extraction by the boiling of dissolved chemicals from plant material (e.g. bark, stems, roots). The process involves mashing or pounding materials and then boiling them in order to extract oils, volatile organic compounds and other chemical substances. A decoction is also the name of the liquid produced.

***Emollient:*** a moisturizer that softens the corneum or outer layer of the epidermis by stimulating rehydration.

***Emulsifier:*** also known as a suspending vehicle or fixative that combines ingredients (that is, stabilizing the volatile components).

***Exfoliant:*** a product made from natural and / or synthetic ingredients to provide a deep cleanse of the face and / or the body by targeting, in particular, the build-up of dead skin cells. Exfoliation results in a healthier looking skin. Exfoliants are removed with water.

***Infusion:*** the process of extraction of properties from plants in a solvent (water, for example), by allowing the substance to remain suspended in the solvent over a period of time (that is, 'steeping'). The liquid produced is also called a 'decoction'.

***Steeping:*** cf. 'infusion'.

***Unguent:*** In antiquity, an unguent took the form of a greasy ointment. As a perfume, an unguent had a liquid base and a scented essence. It could also have additions such as a preservative (salt, for example) and an emulsifier or fixative (such as a gum or resin).

## Appendix 3: Ingredients in the *Medicamina* recipes*

| Recipe | Cleanser | Emollient | Emulsifier |
|---|---|---|---|
| Recipe 1: *ll*.53–68 | Narcissus bulbs | Libyan barley<br>Bitter vetch<br>Hartshorn<br>Tuscan seed | Eggs<br>Gum<br>Honey |
| Recipe 2: *ll*.69–76 | Hydrated soda ash<br>Iris | Lupin seeds<br>Beans | White lead |
| Recipe 3: *ll*.77–82 | *Alcyonea* | Honey | Honey |
| Recipe 4: *ll*.83–90 | Frankincense Natron | Myrrh<br>Honey | Gum<br>Honey |
| Recipe 5: *ll*.91–98 | Fennel<br>Frankincense<br>Salt | Myrrh<br>Rose | Barley water |

* Some ingredients have a dual action, such as frankincense, which can act as a cleanser as well as an emollient. Such ingredients are placed in the category that best reflects their main action in each recipe. In recipes 3 and 4, honey has been categorized as both emollient and emulsifier.

## Appendix 4: Roman weights and measures and equivalents

| Roman unit | relationship to *as* | metric (g) | imperial (oz) |
|---|---|---|---|
| *as / libra / pondus* | 1 | 327.05 | 11.54 |
| *semis / semissis* | 1/2 | 163.53 | 5.77 |
| *triens* | 1/3 | 109.02 | 3.85 |
| *quadrans / teruncius* | 1/4 | 81.76 | 2.88 |
| *sextans* | 1/6 | 54.51 | 1.92 |
| *uncia* | 1/12 | 27.25 | 0.96 |

| Roman unit | relationship to *uncia* | metric (g) | imperial (oz) |
|---|---|---|---|
| *semuncia* | 1/2 | 13.63 | 0.48 |
| *duella* | 1/3 | 9.08 | 0.32 |
| *sicilicus* | 1/4 | 6.81 | 0.24 |
| *sextula* | 1/6 | 4.54 | 0.16 |
| *semisextula* | 1/12 | 2.27 | 0.08 |
| *scripulum* | 1/24 | 1.14 | 0.04 |

# Bibliography

## Ancient texts (Commentaries, editions and translations)

Alexis (1959) *The Fragments of Attic Comedy after Meineke, Bergk, and Kock*, J. M. Edmonds (Leiden: Brill). Vol. 1.
—— (1996) *Alexis: The Fragments: A Commentary*, W. Geoffrey Arnott (Cambridge: Cambridge University Press).
Aristotle (1943) *Generation of Animals*, A. L. Peck (Cambridge, Mass.: Harvard University Press).
—— (1965) *History of Animals*, A. L. Peck (Cambridge, Mass.: Harvard University Press). Books I–III.
—— (1970) *History of Animals*, A. L. Peck (Cambridge, Mass.: Harvard University Press). Books IV–VI.
—— (1991) *History of Animals,* D. M. Balme and A. Gotthelf (Cambridge, Mass.: Harvard University Press). Books VII–X.
Athenaeus (1890) *Athenaei Naucratitae deipnosophistarum libri xv*, G. Kaibel (Leipzig: Teubner). Vol. 3.
Callimachus (1965) *Callimachus I: Fragmenta*, 2nd edn, Rudolph Pfeiffer (Oxford: Oxford University Press).
—— (1953) *Callimachus II: Hymni et Epigrammata*, Rudolph Pfeiffer (Oxford: Oxford University Press).
Celsus (1935–38) *De medicina*, W. G. Spencer (Cambridge, Mass.: Harvard University Press). 3 vols.
Cicero (1991) *Cicero: On Duties*, M. T. Griffin and E. M. Atkins (Cambridge: Cambridge University Press).
Dioscorides (1958) *De materia medica libri quinque / Pedanii Dioscuridis Anazarbei*, M. Wellman (Berlin: Berolini and Weidmannos). 3 vols.
—— (2011) *De materia medica by Pedanius Dioscorides*, 2nd edn, Lily Y. Beck (Hildesheim: Olms-Weidmann).

Galen (1826) *Claudii Galeni Opera Omnia*, D. Carlos Gottlob Kühn (Lipsiae: C. Cnobloch). Vol. XII.

—— (1827) *Claudii Galeni Opera Omnia*, D. Carlos Gottlob Kühn (Lipsiae: C. Cnobloch). Vol. XIV.

*Greek Magical Papyri in Translation, including the Demotic Spells* (1986), H. D. Betz (Chicago: University of Chicago Press).

Horace (2003) *A Commentary on Horace's Epodes*, Lindsay Watson (Oxford: Oxford University Press).

Juvenal (2014) *Juvenal Satire 6*, Lindsay Watson and Patricia Watson (Cambridge: Cambridge University Press).

Lucilius (1967) *Remains of Old Latin. Vol. III*, revised edn, E. H. Warmington (Cambridge, Mass.: Harvard University Press).

Martial (1993) *Epigrams*, D. R. Shackleton Bailey (Cambridge, Mass.: Harvard University Press). 3 vols.

Nicander (1953) *Nicander: The Poems and Poetical Fragments*, A. S. F. Gow and A. F. Scholfield (Cambridge: Cambridge University Press).

Ovid (1727) *P. Ovidii Nasonis opera Omnia* cum integris Micylli, Ciofani et Dan. Heinsii notis et Nic. Heinsii curis secundis, cura et studio Petri Burmanni (Amsterdam: R. et J. Westenios et G. Smith). Vol. 1.

—— (1881) *P. Ovidii Nasonis libellus De medicamine faciei*, A. Kunz (Vienna: Vindobonae).

—— (1955) *P. Ovidi Nasonis Amores*, 2nd edn, F. Munari (Florence: La Nuova Italia).

—— (1958) E. J. Kenney, 'Notes on Ovid', *Classical Quarterly* 8: 54–66.

—— (1961) E. J. Kenney, 'Review', W. Lenz, *Ovid: Heilmittel gegen die Liebe. Die Pflege des weiblichen Gesichts Lateinisch und Deutsch*, *Gnomon* 33: 577–81.

—— (1962) *Ovid II: The Art of Love and Other Poems*, J. H. Mozley (Cambridge, Mass.: Harvard University Press).

—— (1965) G. P. Goold, 'Amatoria Critica', *Harvard Studies in Classical Philology* 69: 1–107.

—— (1965) *Il Codice Hamilton 471 Di Ovidio (Ars Amatoria, Remedia Amoris, Amores)*, F. Munari (Rome: Storia e Letteratura).

—— (1965) *Remedia Amoris; Medicamina Faciei*, F. W. Lenz (Turin: Paravia).

—— (1973) *Amores Book 1*, J. A. Barsby (Oxford: Clarendon Press).

—— (1977) *Ars Amatoria Book I*, A. S. Hollis (Oxford: Clarendon Press).

—— (1977) *Ovid I: Heroides and Amores*, 2nd edn, G. Showerman and G. P. Goold (Cambridge, Mass.: Harvard University Press).

—— (1979) *Ovid II: The Art of Love and Other Poems*, 2nd edn, J. H. Mozley and G. P. Goold (Cambridge, Mass.: Harvard University Press).

—— (1979) *Remedia Amoris*, A. A. R. Henderson (Edinburgh: Scottish Academic Press).

—— (1980) A. A. R. Henderson, 'Notes on the Text of Ovid's *Remedia*', *Classical Quarterly* 30: 159–73.

—— (1983) *Ovid: The Erotic Poems*, Peter Green (Harmondsworth: Penguin).

—— (1985) *I cosmetici delle donne*, Gianpiero Rosati (Italy: Marsilio).

—— (1987) *Amores Vol. I. Text and Prolegomena*, J. C. McKeown (Liverpool: Liverpool Classical Press).

—— (1989) *Amores Vol. II. A Commentary on Book One*, J. C. McKeown (Leeds: Francis Cairns).

—— (1995) *P. Ovidi Nasonis: Amores, Medicamina Faciei Femineae, Ars Amatoria, Remedia Amoris*, 2nd edn, E. J. Kenney (Oxford: Oxford University Press).

—— (2003) *Ars Amatoria Book 3*, Roy K. Gibson (Cambridge: Cambridge University Press).

—— (2004) *The Erotic Poems*, Peter Green (Harmondsworth: Penguin).

—— (2004) E. J. Kenney, 'Review', Antonio Ramírez de Verger, *Ovidius. Carmina Amatoria*, *Bryn Mawr Classical Review*: unpaged.

Philaenis (1972) E. Lobel, '*P.oxy.* n 2891' in E. Lobel (ed.) *The Oxyrhynchus Papyri*, vol. 39 (London: Egypt Exploration Society), 51–4.

Plautus (2011) *Plautus*, Wolfgang de Melo (Cambridge, Mass.: Harvard University Press). Vol. II.

—— (2011) *Plautus*, Wolfgang de Melo (Cambridge, Mass.: Harvard University Press). Vol. III.

Pliny (1938–62) *Natural History*, Harris Rackham, W. H. S. Jones, and D. E. Eichholz (Cambridge, Mass.: Harvard University Press). 10 vols.

Propertius (2007) *Sexti Properti Elegos*, S. J. Heyworth (Oxford: Clarendon Press).

Scribonius (1983) *Compositiones*, Sergio Sconocchia (Leipzig: Teubner).

Seneca (1935) *Seneca: Moral Essays*, John W. Basore (Cambridge, Mass.: Harvard University Press). Vol. III.

Theophrastus (1916) *Enquiry into Plants*, Arthur F. Hort (Cambridge, Mass.: Harvard University Press). Vol. I.

—— (1916) *Enquiry into Plants* (including *On Odours* and *Weather Signs*), Arthur F. Hort (Cambridge, Mass.: Harvard University Press). Vol. II.

Virgil (1988) *Virgil: Georgics. Vol. 1: Books I–II*, Richard F. Thomas (Cambridge: Cambridge University Press).

—— (1994) *Georgics*, R. A. B. Mynors (Oxford: Oxford University Press).

## Modern texts

Acosta-Hughes, Benjamin (2009) 'Ovid and Callimachus: Rewriting the Master' in Peter E. Knox (ed.) *A Companion to Ovid* (Oxford: Wiley-Blackwell). 236–51.

Adams, J. N. (1982) *The Latin Sexual Vocabulary* (London: Duckworth).

Barchiesi, A. (1988) 'Ovid the Censor', *American Journal of Ancient History* 13: 96–105.

Balsdon, J. P. V. D. (1962) *Roman Women: Their History and Habits* (London: Bodley Head).

Barel, André O., Marc Paye and Howard I. Maibach (eds) (2014) *Handbook of Cosmetic Science and Technology*, 4th edn (Basel: Marcel Dekker).

Barini, C. (1958) *Ornatus Muliebris: i gioielli e le antiche romane* (Torino: Loescher).

Bartman, Elizabeth (2001) 'Hair and the Artifice of Roman Female Adornment', *American Journal of Archaeology* 105: 1–25.

Barton, Carlin (2002) 'Being in the Eyes: Shame and Sight in Ancient Rome' in David Fredrick (ed.) *The Roman Gaze: Vision, Power, and the Body* (Baltimore: Johns Hopkins University Press). 216–35.

Bartsch, Shadi (2006) *The Mirror of the Self: Sexuality, Self-Knowledge, and the Gaze in the Early Roman Empire* (Chicago: University of Chicago Press).

Ben-Yehoshua, Shimshon, Carole Borowitz and Lumír Ondřej Hanuš (2012) 'Frankincense, Myrrh, and Balm of Gilead: Ancient Spices of Southern Arabia and Judea' in Jules Janick (ed.) *Horticultural Reviews Volume 39* (Oxford: Wiley-Blackwell). 1–76.

Benediktson, D. Thomas (1985) 'Pictorial Art and Ovid's *Amores*', *Quaderni Urbinati di Cultura Classica* 20: 111–20.

Berman, Kathleen (1972) 'Some Propertian Imitations in Ovid's *Amores*', *Classical Philology* 67: 170–7.

Bertman, Stephen (1989) 'The Ashes and the Flame: Passion and Aging in Classical Poetry', in Thomas M. Falkner and Judith de Luce (eds) *Old Age in Greek and Latin Literature* (Albany: State University of New York Press). 157–71.

Bhishagratna, Kaviraj Kunja Lal (ed.) (1907; 2010) *An English Translation of the Sushruta Samhita, Based on Original Sanskrit Text* (USA: Nabu Press).

Blanco-Dávila, F. (2000) 'Beauty and the Body: The Origins of Cosmetics', *Plastic & Reconstructive Surgery* 105: 1196–1204.

Bonfante, Larissa and Judith Lynn Sebesta (eds) (1994) *The World of Roman Costume* (Wisconsin: University of Wisconsin Press).

Booth, J. (1996) 'Tibullus 1.8 and 1.9: A Tale in Two Poems', *Museum Helveticum* 53: 232–47.

Bowditch, P. Lowell (2012) 'Roman Love Elegy and the Eros of Empire' in Barbara K. Gold (ed.) *A Companion to Roman Love Elegy* (New Jersey: Wiley-Blackwell). 119–33.

Boyd, Barbara W. (1997) *Ovid's Literary Loves: Influence and Innovation in the Amores* (Ann Arbor: University of Michigan Press).

Bradley, Mark (2009) *Colour and Meaning in Ancient Rome* (Cambridge: Cambridge University Press).

Brendel, Otto (1970) 'The Scope and Temperament of Erotic Art in the Greco-Roman World' in T. Bowie et al. (eds) *Studies in Erotic Art* (New York: Basic Books). 3–107.

Broer, P. N. S., M. Levine and S. Juran (2014) 'Plastic Surgery: Quo Vadis? Current Trends and Future Projections of Aesthetic Plastic Surgical Procedures in the United States', *Plastic & Reconstructive Surgery* 133: 293–302.

Brunelle, Christopher (2005) 'Ovid's Satirical Remedies' in Ronnie Ancona and Ellen Greene (eds) *Gendered Dynamics in Latin Love Poetry* (Baltimore: Johns Hopkins University Press). 141–58.

Burlando, Bruno and Laura Cornara (2013) 'Honey in dermatology and skin care: a review', *Journal of Cosmetic Dermatology* 12: 306–13.

Cameron, Alan (1968) 'The First Edition of the *Amores*', *Classical Quarterly* 62: 320–33.

Casali, Sergio (2006) 'The Art of Making Oneself Hated: Rethinking (Anti-) Augustanism in Ovid's *Ars Amatoria*' in Roy K. Gibson, Steven Green and Alison Sharrock (eds) *The Art of Love: Bimillennial Essays on Ovid's Ars Amatoria and Remedia Amoris* (Oxford: Oxford University Press). 216–34.

Cilliers, L. and F. P. Retief (2008) 'Bees, Honey and Health in Antiquity', *Akroterion* 53: 7–19.

Cioccoloni, Francesca (2006) '*Medicamina faciei femineae*: l'ironica polemica di Ovidio rispetto al motivo propagandistico augusteo della *restitutio* dell'età dell'oro', *Latomus* 65: 97–107.

Claassen, Jo-Marie (2008) *Ovid Revisited: The Poet in Exile* (London: Duckworth).

Cleland, Liza, Glenys Davies and Lloyd Llewellyn-Jones (2008) *Greek and Roman Dress from A to Z* (London: Routledge).

Cokayne, Karen (2003) *Experiencing Old Age in Rome* (London: Routledge).

Culham, Phyllis (1982) 'The "Lex Oppia"', *Latomus* 41: 786–93.

d'Ambrosio, Antonio (2001) *Women and Beauty in Pompeii* (Italy: L'ERMA di BRETSCHNEIDER).

Damer, Erika Zimmermann (2014) 'Gender Reversals and Intertextuality in Tibullus', *Classical World* 107: 493–514.

Davis, Peter (1999) 'Ovid's *Amores*: A Political Reading', *Classical Philology* 94.4: 431–49.

—— (2006) *Ovid and Augustus: A political reading of Ovid's erotic poems* (London: Duckworth).

Dewar, Michael (2008) 'Spinning the *Trabea*: Consular Robes and Propaganda in the Panegyrics of Claudian' in Jonathon Edmonson and Alison Keith (eds) *Roman Dress and the Fabrics of Roman Culture* (Toronto: University of Toronto Press). 217–37.

Dirckx, John H. (1980) 'Ovid's dermatologic formulary', *The American Journal of Dermatopathology* 2: 327–32.

Downing, Eric (1999) 'Anti-Pygmalion: The Praeceptor in *Ars Amatoria*, Book 3' in James I. Porter (ed.) *Constructions of the Classical Body* (Michigan: Michigan University Press). 235–52.

Drinkwater, M. O. (2013) '*Militia amoris*: Fighting in love's army' in Thea S. Thorsen (ed.) *The Cambridge Companion to Latin Love Elegy* (Cambridge: Cambridge University Press). 194–206.

Du Quesnay, Ian (2012) 'Three Problems in Poem 66' in Ian Du Quesnay and Tony Woodman (eds) *Catullus: Poems, Books, Readers* (Cambridge: Cambridge University Press). 153–83.

Edmonds II, Radcliffe G. (2013) 'Bewitched, Bothered and Bewildered: Erotic Magic in the Greco-Roman World' in Thomas K. Hubbard (ed.) *A Companion to Greek and Roman Sexualities* (Oxford: Wiley-Blackwell). 282–96.

Edmondson, Jonathan and Alison Keith (eds) (2008) *Roman Dress and the Fabrics of Roman Culture* (Toronto: University of Toronto Press).

Edwards, Catharine (2002) *The Politics of Immorality in Ancient Rome* (Cambridge: Cambridge University Press).

Eidinow, J. S. C. (1993) 'A Note on Ovid *Ars Amatoria* 1.117–19', *American Journal of Philology* 114: 413–17.

Evershed, R. P. et al. (2004) 'Formulation of a Roman Cosmetic', *Nature* 432: 35–6.

Fagan, Garrett G. (1999) *Bathing in Public in the Roman World* (Ann Arbor: University of Michigan Press).

Falkner, Thomas M. (1996) *The Poetics of Old Age in Greek Epic, Lyric and Tragedy* (Oklahoma: University of Oklahoma Press).

Falkner, Thomas M. and Judith de Luce (eds) *Old Age in Greek and Latin Literature* (Albany: State University of New York Press).

Faraone, Christopher A. (1999) *Ancient Greek Love Magic* (USA: Harvard University Press).

Faraone, Christopher A. and Dirk Obbink (eds) (1991) *Magika Hiera: Ancient Greek Magic and Religion* (Oxford: Oxford University Press).

Fitton Brown, A. (1985) 'The Unreality of Ovid's Tomitan Exile', *LCM* 10.2: 18–22.

Forbes, R. J. (1965) *Studies in Ancient Roman Technology Vol. III* (Leiden: Brill).

Fränkel, Hermann (1945) *Ovid: A Poet Between Worlds* (Berkeley: University of California Press).

Gale, Monica R. (2000) *Virgil on the Nature of Things: The Georgics, Lucretius and the Didactic Tradition* (Cambridge: Cambridge University Press).

García, Luis Rivero (1995) 'On a Passage of Ovid (*Med.* 27-36)', *Mnemosyne* 48: 285-91.

Gibson, Roy K. (2006) 'Ovid, Augustus, and the Politics of Moderation in *Ars Amatoria* 3' in Roy K. Gibson, Steven Green and Alison Sharrock (eds) *The Art of Love: Bimillennial Essays on Ovid's Ars Amatoria and Remedia Amoris* (Oxford: Oxford University Press). 121-42.

—— (2007) *Excess and Restraint: Propertius, Horace, and Ovid's Ars Amatoria. BICS, Suppl. 89* (London: Institute of Classical Studies).

Goold, G. P. (1983) 'The Cause of Ovid's Exile', *Illinois Classical Studies* 8.1: 94-107.

Green, Peter (1979) '*Ars Gratia Cultus*: Ovid as Beautician', *American Journal of Philology* 100: 381-92.

—— (1982) 'Carmen et Error: πρόφασις and αἰτία in the Matter of Ovid's Exile', *Classical Antiquity* 1.2: 202-20.

Green, Steven J. (2006) 'Lessons in Love: Fifty Years of Scholarship on the *Ars Amatoria* and *Remedia Amoris*' in Roy Gibson, Stephen Green and Alison Sharrock (eds) *The Art of Love: Bimillennial Essays on Ovid's Ars Amatoria and Remedia Amoris* (Oxford: Oxford University Press). 1-20.

Greene, Ellen (1994) 'Sexual Politics in Ovid's *Amores*: 3.4, 3.8, and 3.12', *Classical Philology* 89.4: 344-50.

Griffin, A. H. F. (1981) 'The Ceyx Legend in Ovid, *Metamorphoses*, Book XI', *Classical Quarterly* 31: 147-54.

—— (1991) 'Philemon and Baucis in Ovid's *Metamorphoses*', *Greece & Rome* 38: 62-74.

Griffin, Jasper (1976) 'Augustan Poetry and the Life of Luxury', *Journal of Roman Studies* 66: 87-105.

Grillet, B (1975) *Les femmes et les fards dans l'Antiquité grecque* (Lyon: Centre National de la Recherche Scientifique).

Gutzwiller, Kathryn (1992) '"Callimachus" Lock of Berenice: Fantasy, Romance, and Propaganda', *American Journal of Philology* 113: 359-85.

Habinek, Thomas (2002) 'Ovid and Empire' in Philip Hardie (ed.) *The Cambridge Companion to Ovid* (Cambridge: Cambridge University Press). 46-61.

Hanson, Ann Ellis (2009) 'A Receptarium from Tebtunis' in I. Andorlini (ed.) *Greek Medical Papyri II* (Firenze: Istituto Papirologico 'G. Vitelli'). 71-103.

Hardie, Philip (2002) *Ovid's Poetics of Illusion* (Cambridge: Cambridge University Press).

—— (2006) '*Lethaeus Amor:* The Art of Forgetting' in Roy Gibson, Stephen Green and Alison Sharrock (eds) *The Art of Love: Bimillennial Essays on Ovid's Ars Amatoria and Remedia Amoris* (Oxford: Oxford University Press). 166–90.

Harlow, Mary (ed.) (2012) *Dress and Identity* (Oxford: Archaeopress).

Hejduk, Julia Dyson (2014) 'Introduction' in *The Offence of Love: Ars Amatoria, Remedia Amoris,* and *Tristia 2. A verse translation* (Madison: The University of Wisconsin Press).

Heldmann, K (1982) 'Ovid über den Pfau: Zum Lobe der Schönheit' *Hermes* 110: 375–80.

Henderson, John (2006) 'In Ovid with Bed (*Ars* 2 and 3)' in Roy Gibson, Stephen Green and Alison Sharrock (eds) *The Art of Love: Bimillennial Essays on Ovid's Ars Amatoria and Remedia Amoris* (Oxford: Oxford University Press). 77–95.

Hendry, Michael (1995) 'Rouge and Crocodile Dung: Notes on Ovid, *Ars* 3.199–200 and 269–270', *Classical Quarterly* 45: 583–8.

Higgins, Reynold (1980) *Greek and Roman Jewellery*, 2nd edn (Berkeley: University of California Press).

Hill, D. (1973) 'The Thessalian Trick', *Rheinisches Museum für Philologie* 116: 221–38.

Hinds, Stephen (1998) *Allusion and Intertext: Dynamics of Appropriation in Roman Poetry* (Cambridge: Cambridge University Press).

—— (2002) 'Landscape and figures: aesthetics of place in the *Metamorphoses* and its tradition' in Philip Hardie (ed.) *The Cambridge Companion to Ovid* (Cambridge: Cambridge University Press). 122–49.

Hodges, Frederick Mansfield (2001) 'The Ideal Prepuce in Ancient Greece and Rome: Male Genital Aesthetics and Their Relation to *Lipodermos*, Circumcision, Foreskin Restoration, and the *Kynodesmē*', *Bulletin of the History of Medicine* 75: 375–405.

Holleman, A. W. J. (1971) 'Ovid and Politics', *Historia: Zeitschrift für Alte Geschichte* 20.4: 458–66.

Holzberg, Niklas (2006) 'Staging the Reader Response: Ovid and His "Contemporary Audience"' in Roy Gibson, Stephen Green and Alison Sharrock (eds) *The Art of Love: Bimillennial Essays on Ovid's Ars Amatoria and Remedia Amoris* (Oxford: Oxford University Press). 40–53.

Howe, Thalia Phillies (1958) 'Linear B and Hesiod's Breadwinners', *Transactions of the American Philological Society* 89: 44–65.

Huskey, S. (2005) 'In Memory of Tibullus: Ovid's Remembrance of Tibullus 1.3 in *Amores* 3.9 and *Tristia* 3.3', *Arethusa* 38: 367–86.

Hunter, Richard (2006) *The Shadow of Callimachus. Studies in the Reception of Hellenistic Poetry at Rome* (Cambridge: Cambridge University Press).

Jahn, P. (1903) 'Eine Prosaquelle Vergils und ihre Umsetzung in Poesie durch den Dichter' *Hermes* 38: 244–64.

James, Sharon L. (2003) *Learned Girls and Male Persuasion: Gender and Reading in Roman Love Elegy* (Berkeley: University of California Press).

Jansen, Laura (2012) 'On the Edge of the Text: Preface and Reader in Ovid's *Amores*', *Helios* 39.1: 1-19.

Johnson, Patricia J. (1997) 'Ovid's Livia in Exile', *Classical World* 90: 403-20.

Jones, C. P. (1987) 'Stigmata: Tattooing and Branding in Graeco-Roman Antiquity', *Journal of Roman Studies* 77: 139-55.

Keith, Alison (2009) 'Sexuality and Gender' in Peter E. Knox (ed.) *A Companion to Ovid* (Oxford: Wiley-Blackwell). 355-69.

—— (2011) (ed.) *Latin Elegy and Hellenistic Epigram. A Tale of Two Genres at Rome* (Newcastle upon Tyne: Cambridge Scholars Publications).

Kennedy, Duncan F. (1997) 'Bluff your way in Didactic: Ovid's *Ars Amatoria* and *Remedia Amoris*', *Arethusa* 33: 159-76.

Keyser, Paul T. and Georgia L. Irby-Massie (eds) (2009) *The Encyclopedia of Ancient Natural Scientists* (London: Routledge).

Khan, H. A. (1966) '*Ovidius Furens*: A Revaluation of *Amores* I.7', *Latomus* 25: 880-94.

Küppers, E. (1981) 'Ovids *Ars Amatoria* und *Remedia Amoris* als Lehrdichtungen', *Aufstieg und Niedergang der römischen Welt* 2.31.4: 2507-51.

Labate, Mario (1984) *L'arte di farsi amare: Modelli culturali e progetto didascalico nell'elegia ovidiana* (Pisa: Giardini).

—— (2006) 'Erotic Aetiology: Romulus, Augustus, and the Rape of the Sabine Women' in Roy Gibson, Stephen Green and Alison Sharrock (eds) *The Art of Love: Bimillennial Essays on Ovid's Ars Amatoria and Remedia Amoris* (Oxford: Oxford University Press). 193-215.

Laca, A., B. Paredes and M. Díaz (2012) 'Lipid-Enriched Egg Yolk Fraction as Ingredient in Cosmetic Emulsions', *Journal of Texture Studies* 43: 12-28.

Langlands, Rebecca (2006) *Sexual Morality in Ancient Rome* (Cambridge: Cambridge University Press).

Lateiner, D. (2005) 'Signifying Names and Other Ominous Accidental Utterances in Classical Historiography', *Greek, Roman and Byzantine Studies* 45: 35-57.

Leary, T. J. (1988a) 'Three Observations on Ovid's *Medicamina* (13-14, 63-4, 87-8)', *Liverpool Classical Monthly* 13: 25-6.

—— (1988b) 'The *Medicamina* Recalled', *Liverpool Classical Monthly* 13: 140-42.

—— (1990) 'That's what little girls are made of: the charms of elegiac women', *Liverpool Classical Monthly* 15: 152-5.

—— (1996) *Martial Book XIV: The Apophoreta* (London: Duckworth).

Lessler, Milton A. (1988) 'Lead and Lead Poisoning from Antiquity to Modern Times', *The Ohio Journal of Science* 88: 78-84.

Levy, Harry (1968) 'Hair!', *Classical World* 62: 135.

Lightfoot, Jane (2009) 'Ovid and Hellenistic Poetry' in Peter E. Knox (ed.) *A Companion to Ovid* (Oxford: Wiley-Blackwell). 219–35.

Lilja, Saara (1965; 1978) *The Roman Elegists' Attitude to Women* (New York: Garland).

—— (1972) *The Treatment of Odours in the Poetry of Antiquity* (Helsinki: Societas Scientiarum Fennica).

Lovén, Lena Larsson (1998) 'LENAM FECIT: woolworking and female *virtus*' in Lena Larsson Lovén and Agneta Strömberg (eds) *Aspects of Women in Antiquity* (Jonsered: Astöms Forlag). 85–95.

Lucas, A (1930) 'Cosmetics, Perfumes, and Incense in Ancient Egypt', *The Journal of Egyptian Archaeology* 16: 41–53.

Lurie, Alison (1981) *The Language of Clothes* (London: Random House).

Majno, Guido (1975) *The Healing Hand: Man and Wound in the Ancient World* (Cambridge, Mass.: Harvard University Press).

Makdisi, Joy, Allison Kutner and Adam Friedman (2014) 'Oats and Skin Health' in YiFang Chu (ed.) *Oats Nutrition and Technology* (Oxford: Wiley-Blackwell). 326–34.

Marmelzat, W. L. (1987) 'History of Dermatologic Surgery from the Beginnings to Late Antiquity', *Clinics in Dermatology* 5: 1–10.

McGinn, T. A. J. (1991) 'Concubinage and the *Lex Iulia* on adultery', *Transactions of the American Philological Association* 121: 335–75.

McGowan, Matthew M. (2009) *Ovid in Exile: Power and Poetic Redress in the Tristia and Epistulae Ex Ponto* (Leiden: Brill).

Miller, Anthony and Miranda Morris (1988) *Plants of Dhofar. The Southern Region of Oman: Traditional, Economic and Medicinal Uses* (Oman: The Office of The Adviser for Conservation of The Environment, Diwan of Royal Court Sultanate of Oman).

Miller, John. F. (1983) 'Callimachus and the *Ars Amatoria*', *Classical Philology* 78.1: 26–34.

—— (1997) 'Lucretian Moments in Ovidian Elegy', *Classical Journal* 92: 384–98.

Miller, Paul Allen (2013) 'The *puella*: accept no substitutions!' in Thea S. Thorsen (ed.) *The Cambridge Companion to Latin Love Elegy* (Cambridge: Cambridge University Press). 166–79.

Milleker, Elizabeth J. (1988) 'The Three Graces on a Roman Relief Mirror', *Metropolitan Museum Journal* 23: 69–81.

Mitsdörffer, W. (1938) 'Vergils Georgica und Theophrast', *Philologus* 93: 449–75.

Morgan, Kathleen (1977) *Ovid's Art of Imitation: Propertius in the Amores* (Leiden: Brill).

Morrison, J. V. (1992) 'Literary Reference and Generic Transgression in Ovid, *Amores* 1.7: Lover, Poet, and *Furor*', *Latomus* 51: 571–89.

Morrison, Wendy A. (2013) 'A Fresh Eye on Familiar Objects: Rethinking Toiletry Sets in Roman Britain', *Oxford Journal of Archaeology* 32: 221–30.
Murgatroyd, P. (1975) '*Militia amoris* and the Roman Elegists', *Latomus* 34: 59–79.
Myers, K. Sara (1996) 'The Poet and the Procuress: The *Lena* in Latin Love Elegy', *Journal of Roman Studies* 86: 1–21.
Myerowitz, Molly (1992) 'The Domestication of Desire: Ovid's *Parva Tabella* and the Theater of Love' in Amy Richlin (ed.) *Pornography and Representation in Greece and Rome* (New York: Oxford University Press). 131–57.
Nelis, Damien P. (2012) 'Callimachus in Verona: Catullus and Alexandrian Poetry' in Ian Du Quesnay and Tony Woodman (eds) *Catullus: Poems, Books, Readers* (Cambridge: Cambridge University Press). 1–28.
Nikolaidis, Anastasios (1994) 'On a Supposed Contradiction in Ovid (*Medicamina Faciei* 18–22 vs. *Ars Amatoria* 3.129–32)', *American Journal of Philology* 115: 97–103.
Norwood, Frances (1963) 'The Riddle of Ovid's *Relegatio*' 58.3: 150–63.
Ogden, Jack (1992) *Ancient Jewellery* (Berkeley: University of California Press).
Olson, Kelly (2002) 'Matrona and Whore: The Clothing of Women in Roman Antiquity', *Fashion Theory* 6: 387–420.
—— (2008a) *Dress and the Roman Woman: Self-Presentation and Society* (London: Routledge).
—— (2008b) 'The Appearance of the Young Roman Girl' in Jonathan Edmondson and Alison Keith (eds) *Roman Dress and the Fabrics of Roman Culture* (Toronto: University of Toronto Press). 139–57.
—— (2009) 'Cosmetics in Roman Antiquity: Substance, Remedy, Poison', *Classical World* 102: 291–310.
Otis, Brooks (1970) *Ovid as an Epic Poet*, 2nd edn (Cambridge: Cambridge University Press).
Papaioannou, Sophia (2006) 'The Poetology of Hairstyling and the Excitement of Hair Loss in Ovid, "Amores" 1,14', *Materiali e discussioni per l'analisi dei testi classici* 83: 45–69.
Parker, Holt N. (1989) 'Another Go at the Text of Philaenis (P. Oxy. 2891)', *Zeitschrift für Papyrologie und Epigraphik* 79: 49–50.
—— (1992) 'Love's Body Anatomized: The Ancient Erotic Handbooks and the Rhetoric of Sexuality' in Amy Richlin (ed.) *Pornography and Representation in Greece and Rome* (New York: Oxford University Press). 90–111.
—— (1997) 'Women Physicians in Greece, Rome, and the Byzantine Empire' in L. R. Furst (ed.) *Women Physicians and Healers: Climbing a Long Hill* (Lexington: University Press of Kentucky). 131–50.

—— (2012) 'Galen and the Girls: Sources for Women Medical Writers Revisited', *Classical Quarterly* 62: 359–86.

Parkin, Tim (2003) *Old Age in the Roman World: A Cultural Social History* (Baltimore: Johns Hopkins University Press).

Potter, David S. (2002) 'Odor and Power in the Roman Empire' in James I. Porter (ed.) *Constructions of the Classical Body* (Ann Arbor: University of Michigan Press). 169–89.

Reed, J. (1997) 'Ovid's Elegy on Tibullus and Its Models', *Classical Philology* 92: 260–9.

Reinhold, Meyer (1970) *History of Purple as a Status Symbol in Antiquity* (Brussels: Latomus).

Richlin, Amy (1984) 'Invective against Women in Roman Satire', *Arethusa* 17: 67–80.

—— (1995) 'Making Up a Woman: The Face of Roman Gender' in Howard Eilberg-Schwartz and Wendy Doniger (eds) *Off With Her Head! The Denial of Women's Identity in Myth, Religion, and Culture* (Berkeley: University of California Press). 185–213.

Riddle, John M (1997) *Eve's Herbs: A History of Contraception and Abortion in the West* (Cambridge, Mass.: Harvard University Press).

Rimell, Victoria (2005) 'Facing Facts: Ovid's *Medicamina* through the Looking Glass' in Ronnie Ancona and Ellen Greene (eds) *Gendered Dynamics in Latin Love Poetry* (Baltimore: Johns Hopkins University Press). 177–205.

—— (2006) *Ovid's Lovers: Desire, Difference and the Poetic Imagination* (Cambridge: Cambridge University Press).

Rinzler, C. A. (ed.) (2009) *The Encyclopedia of Cosmetic and Plastic Surgery* (New York: Facts on File).

Rosati, Gianpiero (2006) 'The Art of *Remedia Amoris:* Unlearning to Love?' in Roy Gibson, Stephen Green and Alison Sharrock (eds) *The Art of Love: Bimillennial Essays on Ovid's Ars Amatoria and Remedia Amoris* (Oxford: Oxford University Press). 143–65.

Ross, David O. (1969) *Style and Tradition in Catullus* (Cambridge, Mass.: Harvard University Press).

Saiko, Maren (2005) *Cura dabit faciem: Kosmetik im Altertum* (Trier: Wissenschaftlicher Verlag).

Salzman-Mitchell, Patricia (2008) 'Snapshots of a Love Affair: *Amores* 1.5 and the Program of Elegiac Narrative' in Genevieve Liveley and Patricia Salzman-Mitchell (eds) *Latin Elegy and Narratology: Fragments of Story* (Ohio: The Ohio State University). 34–47.

Scarborough, J. (1996) 'Drugs and Medicines in the Roman World', *Expedition* 38: 38–51.

—— (2008) 'Sextius Niger' in Paul T. Keyser and Georgia L. Irby-Massie (eds) *The Encyclopedia of Ancient Natural Scientists* (London: Routledge). 738–9.

Scheid, John (2007) 'Sacrifices for Gods and Ancestors' in Jörg Rüpke (ed.) *A Companion to Roman Religion* (Oxford: Blackwell) 263–74.

Sebesta, Judith Lynn (1994) '*Tunica Ralla, Tunica Spissa*: The Colors and Textiles of Roman Costume' in Larissa Bonfante and Judith Lynn Sebesta (eds) *The World of Roman Costume* (Wisconsin: University of Wisconsin Press). 65–76.

—— (1997) 'Women's Costume and Feminine Civic Morality in Augustan Rome', *Gender & History* 9: 529–41.

Segal, Charles (1969) *Landscape in Ovid's Metamorphoses. A study in the transformations of a literary symbol* (Wiesbaden: F. Steiner Verlag).

Shapiro, Arthur K. and Elaine Shapiro (1997) *The Powerful Placebo: From Ancient Priest to Modern Physician* (Baltimore: Johns Hopkins University Press).

Sharrock, Alison (1994) *Seduction and Repetition in Ovid's Ars Amatoria II* (Oxford: Oxford University Press).

—— (2006) 'Love in Parentheses: Digression and Narrative Hierarchy in Ovid's Erotodidactic Poems' in Roy Gibson, Stephen Green and Alison Sharrock (eds) *The Art of Love: Bimillennial Essays on Ovid's Ars Amatoria and Remedia Amoris* (Oxford: Oxford University Press). 23–39.

Shear, T. Leslie (1936) 'Psimythion' in *Classical Studies Presented to Edward Capps on his Seventieth Birthday* (Princeton: Princeton University Press). 314–17.

Shumka, Leslie (2008) 'Designing Women: The Representation of Women's Toiletries on Funerary Monuments in Roman Italy' in Jonathan Edmondson and Alison Keith (eds) *Roman Dress and the Fabrics of Roman Culture* (Toronto: University of Toronto Press). 172–91.

Singer, Armand E. and Mary W. Singer (1950) 'An Ancient Dentifrice', *Classical Weekly* 43: 217–18.

Skinner, Marilyn (1982) 'The Contents of Caelius' "Pyxis"', *Classical World* (74): 243–5.

Solodow, J. B. (1977) 'Ovid's Ars Amatoria: The Lover as Cultural Ideal', *Wiener Studien* 11: 106–127.

Spier, Jeffrey (1992) *Ancient Gems and Finger Rings: Catalogue of the Collection* (California: Getty Publications).

St. Clair, Archer (2003) *Carving as Craft: Palatine East and the Greco-Roman Bone and Ivory Carving Tradition* (Baltimore: Johns Hopkins University Press).

Stephens, Janet (2008) 'Ancient Roman Hairdressing: on (hair)pins and needles', *Journal of Roman Archaeology* 21: 111–32.

Stewart, Susan (2007) *Cosmetics and Perfumes in the Roman World* (Stroud, UK: Tempus).

—— (2012) 'Cosmetics and Perfumes in the Roman World: A Glossary' in Mary Harlow (ed.) *Dress and Identity* (Oxford: Archaeopress). 109–16.

Stirrup, B. E. (1973) 'Irony in Ovid *Amores* I.7', *Latomus* 32: 824–31.

Stout, Ann (1994) 'Jewellery as a Symbol of Status in the Roman Empire' in Larissa Bonfante and Judith Lynn Sebesta (eds) *The World of Roman Costume* (Wisconsin: University of Wisconsin Press). 77–100.

Stratton, Kimberly B. (2014) 'Magic, Abjection, and Gender' in Kimberly B. Stratton and Dayna S. Kalleres (eds) *Daughters of Hecate: Women and Magic in the Ancient World* (Oxford: Oxford University Press). 152–80.

Tarrant, Richard (2013) 'Ovid and ancient literary history' in Philip Hardie (ed.) *The Cambridge Companion to Ovid* (Cambridge: Cambridge University Press). 13–33.

Taylor, R, (2008) *The Moral Mirror of Roman Art* (Cambridge: Cambridge University Press).

Thomas, Richard F. (1987) 'Prose into Poetry: Tradition and Meaning in Virgil's *Georgics*', *Harvard Studies in Classical Philology* 91: 229–60.

Toner, J. P. (1995) *Leisure and Ancient Rome* (Cambridge: Polity Press).

Toohey, Peter (2013) *Epic Lessons: An Introduction to Ancient Didactic Poetry* (London: Routledge).

Treggiari, Susan (1976) 'Jobs for Women', *American Journal of Ancient History* 1: 48–77.

Tsantsanoglou, K. (1973) 'The memoirs of a lady from Samos', *Zeitschrift für Papyrologie und Epigraphik* 12: 183–95.

Tupet, Anne-Marie (1976) *La magie dans la poésie latine* (Paris: Belles Lettres).

—— (1986) 'Rites Magiques dans L'Antiquité Romaine', *Aufstieg und Niedergang der römischen Welt* 16: 2591–675.

Veyne, Paul (1988) *Roman Erotic Elegy: Love, Poetry and the West* (Chicago: University of Chicago Press).

Volk, Katharina (2006) '*Ars Amatoria Romana*: Ovid on Love as a Cultural Construct' in Roy K. Gibson, Steven Green and Alison Sharrock (eds) *The Art of Love: Bimillennial Essays on Ovid's Ars Amatoria and Remedia Amoris* (Oxford: Oxford University Press). 235–51.

Vout, Caroline (1996) 'The Myth of the Toga: Understanding the History of Roman Dress', *Greece and Rome* 43: 204–20.

Walton, F. T. (1946) 'My Lady's Toilet', *Greece & Rome* 15: 68–73.

Watson, Patricia. A. (1982) 'Ovid and *Cultus*: Ars Amatoria 3.113–28', *Transactions of the American Philological Association* 112: 237–44.

—— (1983) '*Puella* and *Virgo*', *Glotta* 61: 119–43.

—— (1993) 'Stepmothers and *Hippomanes*: Georgics 3.282f', *Latomus* 52: 842–7.

—— (2001) 'Parody and Subversion in Ovid's *Medicamina Faciei Femineae*', *Mnemosyne* 54: 457–71.
—— (2002) '*Praecepta Amoris*: Ovid's Didactic Elegy' in Barbara Weiden Boyd (ed.) *Brill's Companion to Ovid* (Leiden: Brill). 141–66.
—— (2007) 'A *Matrona* Makes Up: Fantasy and Reality in Juvenal, Sat. 6,457–507', *Rheinisches Museum für Philologie* 150: 375–95.
Wheeler, A. L. (1934) *Catullus and the Traditions of Ancient Poetry* (Berkeley: University of California Press).
Wildberger, J. (1998) *Ovids Schule der 'elegischen' Liebe: Erotodidaxe und Psychagogie in der Ars Amatoria* (Frankfurt: Peter Lang).
Wilkinson, L. P. (1955) *Ovid Recalled* (Cambridge: Cambridge University Press).
Williams, Gareth (1994) *Banished Voices: Readings in Ovid's Exile Poetry* (Cambridge: Cambridge University Press).
Wilner, Ortha L. (1931) 'Roman Beauty Culture', *Classical Journal* 27: 26–38.
Winkler, John J. (1991) 'The Constraints of Eros' in Christopher A. Faraone and Dirk Obbink (eds) *Magika Hiera: Ancient Greek Magic and Religion* (Oxford: Oxford University Press). 214–43.
Winter, Ruth (2009) *A Consumer's Dictionary of Cosmetic Ingredients*, 7th edn (London: Random House).
Wood, Susan E. (2000) *Imperial Women: A Study in Public Images, 40 BC–AD 68* (Leiden: Brill).
Wray, David (2009) 'Ovid's Catullus and the Neoteric Moment in Roman Poetry' in Peter E. Knox (ed.) *A Companion to Ovid* (Oxford: Wiley-Blackwell). 252–64.
Wyke, Maria (1994) 'Woman in the Mirror: The Rhetoric of Adornment in the Roman World' in Léonie J. Archer, Susan Fischler and Maria Wyke (eds) *Women in Ancient Societies: An Illusion in the Night* (London: Macmillan). 134–51.
Zanda, Emanuela (2011) *Fighting Hydra-like Luxury: Sumptuary Regulation in the Roman Republic* (London: Bloomsbury).
Zanker, Paul (1990) *The Power and Images in the Age of Augustus*, trans. Alan Shapiro (USA: University of Michigan Press).
Zetzel, James E. G. (1996) 'Poetic Baldness and Its Cure' *Materiali e discussioni per l'analisi dei testi classici* 36: 73–100.

# Index of Passages

ALEXIS, *Isostasion*, Fragment 103   2, 5, 17, 35
APICIUS, *The Art of Cooking* 5.4   68
APULEIUS
   *Metamorphoses*
      1.3   57
      3.21ff   129
ARISTOPHANES, *Clouds* 746–757   57
ARISTOTLE
   *History of Animals*
      572a-b   56
      577a   56
      616a   72
ATHENAEUS, 568a-d   2

CALLIMACHUS
   *Epigram* 6   30
   *Fragment* 110   30
   *Iambus* 4   38 n.24
CATULLUS
   1.4   23
   2.1   50
   3.4   50
   6.1   50
   35.1   51
   37.20   119
   39.17–21   119
   45.24   50
   51.2   112
   64.61–68   93
   66   30
   67   39 n.31
   68.70   60
   69.5   116
   74.2   50
CELSUS
   2.12   61
   2.33   61, 64
   3.20   64
   5.5   64, 76
   5.6   65, 76
   5.15   65, 70, 78
   5.16   64, 67
   5.17   76
   5.28   68
   7.8   1
   7.10   1
   7.12   1
CICERO
   *Against Catiline* 2.22–23   53
   *Against Verres* 2.5.31   53
   *On Duties*
      1.4ff   134
      1.17   134
      1.24   134
      1.28   134
      1.130   133
CLAUDIAN, 'Epithalamium of Honorius and Maria'   120
*CORPUS INSCRIPTIONUM LATINARUM*
   6.9730   92
   11.1471   93

DIOSCORIDES
   1.1   70
   1.64   77
   1.68   76, 78
   2.4   118
   2.74   122
   2.77   123
   2.109   68
   2.173   56
   3.70   78
   4.158   65
   5.88   69
   5.118   72

GALEN
   12.47–48   81
   12.308   81
   12.403–404   113

12.404   113
12.416   32
12.421   72
12.432–435   8
12.434–435   8
12.445–446   8
12.449–450   8
14.422–423   64
14.536   72
GREEK ANTHOLOGY
   5.21   58
   5.28   58
   5.76   58
   5.103   58
   5.112   58
   5.204   58
   11.67   58
   11.69   58
GREEK MAGICAL PAPYRI, XII:
   401–444   81

HIPPOCRATES (HIPPOCRATIC
   CORPUS)
   Diseases of Women
     1.106   8
     2.189   9
HOMER
   Iliad
     8.103   58
     14.166ff   9
     19.336   58
     23.623   58
   Odyssey, 11.196   58
HOMERIC HYMN TO APHRODITE,
   ll.218–238   58
HORACE
   Epistles, 1.2.54   65
   Epodes
     2.41–42   50
     5   55
     5.45–46   57
     8   58
     8.3   119
     12   58
     12.1–20   35
     12.5   116
     12.10–11   6
     17   55
     17.29   56

   Satires
     1.2.123–124   6
     1.8   55

ISIDORUS
   Etymologiae
     19.31   110
     20.13   93

JUVENAL
   2.93   120
   6.457–507   6
   6.463   7
   6.487–505   92
   6.595   128

LIVY
   1.10–14   50
   34.7   10
LUCAN
   6.461–484   56
   6.499–506   57
LUCIAN, The Lover of Lies
   ll.11–13   56
LUCILIUS, Fragment
   605–606   56

MARTIAL
   Epigrams
     1.72   70
     1.96   53
     2.17   92
     2.29.9   2, 120
     2.41.11–12   6, 70
     2.66   92
     3.74   53, 117
     6.57   113
     6.64.26   2
     6.74   113
     7.25   70
     8.33.22   2, 120
     10.56.6   2
     10.90   117
     12.23   113
     12.32.21–22   117
     12.43.4   40 n.35
   On the Spectacles
     3.9   95
     14.26   95

# Index of Passages

NICANDER
   *Alexipharmaca* 43  78
   *Theriaca* 94  78

OVID
   *Amores*
     1.1  19, 30
     1.2  19
     1.5  19, 86
     1.5.10  60
     1.8  112
     1.8.21ff  38
     1.8.39–40  50
     1.8.13–14  128
     1.9  19
     1.9.37–38  93
     1.10.35  54
     1.11  86, 92
     **1.14**  83–96
     1.14.1  29, 49
     1.14.9–12  114
     1.14.19–20  111
     1.14.37–38  10
     1.14.41  112
     1.15.9–30  28
     2.1  28
     2.4  112
     2.4.15–16  50
     2.5.13ff  38
     2.6  86
     2.7  92
     2.8  19, 86, 92
     2.8.1  91
     2.9  19
     2.10.5  18
     2.11  86
     2.12  86
     2.12.1–4  38 n.17
     2.12.21–24  50
     2.13  38 n.21, 86
     2.13.24  75
     2.14  38 n.21
     2.16  90
     2.17  86
     2.18  28
     2.18.29  60
     2.19  19, 86
     2.19.46  87
     2.19.57  87
     3.1  86
     3.1.7–10  22–23
     3.1.7–20  28
     3.3.5  60
     3.3.25  60
     3.4  18, 19
     3.4.37–42  18
     3.7  19, 86
     3.7.1  18
     3.8  19, 28
     3.8.2  60
     3.8.61  50
     3.9  19
     3.12  86
   *Ars Amatoria*
     1.1–4  31
     1.7  60
     1.31–34  20, 37 n.14
     1.33–34  31
     1.101–134  50, 112
     1.505  88
     1.505–506  117
     **1.505–524**  131–135
     1.509  48
     1.518  88
     1.527–541  93
     2.99ff  55
     2.100  56
     2.102  56
     2.215–216  10
     2.273  60
     2.599–600  20
     2.657–666  32
     2.679–680  33
     2.745–746  31
     3.17–18  111
     3.43  138
     3.57–58  20
     3.99–100  106
     3.101  48
     3.101–120  107
     3.101–208  127
     **3.101–250**  97–124, 126
     3.102  48
     3.103  48
     3.105  48
     3.107  48
     3.107–108  107
     3.113–120  109

3.113–126   109
3.121–126   109
3.123–126   109
3.127   48
3.127–128   18
3.129–134   16, 52
3.133   88
3.133–250   107
3.134   110
3.135–136   10
3.135–160   91
3.137–168   51
3.141   88
3.145   88
3.153   88
3.153–154   92
3.157ff   93
3.161   88
3.163–168   95
3.202   1
3.205   23, 38 n.18
3.207   139
3.209–234   17, 127
3.209–250   123
3.211–218   7
3.217   48, 123
3.219   17
3.221   17
3.223–224   17
3.224   94
3.225   48
3.234   48
3.235   88
3.235–236   127
3.235–250   51
3.239f   92
3.243   88
3.246   88
3.247–250   127
3.251–380   107
3.255–256   48
3.255–286   4
3.261   48
3.270   81
3.281–282   118, 133
3.333   51
3.361   20
3.380   106
3.381–498   107

3.401   94
3.483   20
3.499   107
3.499–500   107
3.514   133
3.515   133, 140
3.516   133, 140
3.517–518   133
3.519–520   133
3.521   133
3.522   133
3.611–658   21, 37 n.12
3.613–616   20
3.690   115
3.769–788   32
3.783ff   93
*Epistles*
1.4   139
1.5.22   54
3.1.93–94   59
3.3.51–52   37 n.14
*Fasti*
2.9   21
2.461   94
4.139   115
5.309   94
*Heroides*
3   116
12   55
13   111
15.216   60
17.173–174   58
**Medicamina**
*ll*.**1–100**   41–82
*l*.10   26, 49, 111
*l*.37   94
*l*.51   23
*ll*.1–50   23
*ll*.3–24   107
*ll*.7–10   26, 109, 135
*ll*.11–16   50, 107
*ll*.23–24   18
*ll*.23–26   18
*ll*.25–26   18
*ll*.45–48   10
*ll*.99–100   119
*Metamorphoses*
1.564   94
1.722–723   55

2.216–217   54
2.349   60
2.754–755   127
4.300–301   90
4.327   54
5.236–249   116
6.78–79   127
6.412–674   128
6.661   139
7.1–4   128
7.198–202   56
7.207–209   57
7.262   128
10.243–297   123
10.252   123
10.298–502   76
11.92   139
11.410–748   74
15.385   55
Book 7   55
Book 14   55
*Remedia Amores*
  39–40   33
  45–46   34
  75–78   22
  249–290   55
  301–302   52
  325–342   4, 35
  343–344   127
  **343–356**   17, 121, 125–130
  347   139
  351   80
  351–356   7
  355   128
  361–396   21
  377–378   34
  389–392   21
  429–432   35
  437–440   34
  757   51
*Tristia*
  2.207   31
  2.212   37 n.14
  2.346   37 n.14
  2.447–448   39 n.28
  2.471–490   24
  2.491   24
  2.493   24
  2.521–528   33

2.527   94
5.4.21–28   59
OXYRHYNCHUS PAPYRI, 39.2891   32

PETRONIUS
  *Satyricon*
    110   120
    126   120
PLATO, *Gorgias* 513a   57
PLAUTUS
  *Epidicus*, ll. 223–224   113
  *The Haunted House*
    l.289   49
    ll.258–264   4
    ll.273–278   4
PLINY THE ELDER
  3.70   78
  9.54   52
  9.114   6
  12.51–65   75
  12.61   78
  12.63   75
  13.9   78
  13.20–25   6
  14.123   117
  15.87   88
  16.62   90
  16.71   67
  16.180   88
  18.61   67
  20.4   67
  20.20   61, 64
  20.23   67
  20.26   61
  20.43   78
  20.81   61
  20.195   78
  21.123   120
  21.129   61
  21.142   116
  21.143   70
  22.3–4   115
  22.151   64
  22.153   88
  22.154–57   68
  22.188   78
  22.201   78
  22.246   78
  23.94   78

24.106   65
24.154   77
26.164   88, 117
27.53   78
28.28   56, 80
28.81   32
28.163   120
28.178   64
28.178-79   117
28.184-185   80
28.185   123
28.187   64
28.191   88
28.233   64
28.241   64, 123
28.249   117
28.255   117
29.35-37   122
29.36   129
29.46   118
29.126   120
30.10   67
30.132-134   117
30.134   120
31.117   118
32.65   118
32.67   88
32.86-87   72
32.87   68
32.136   117
33.102   121
33.102-103   120
33.109   95
34.167   68
34.175   69
35.36   94
35.185   116
35.194   88
36.154   117
36.156   118
Book 37   52
PLUTARCH, *Romulus* 19-24   50
PROPERTIUS
   1.1   55
   1.2.1   29
   1.2.7-8   6
   1.3.1-8   93
   1.9.1   29
   1.16   39 n.31

2.18.23-28   7
2.32   50
2.34.27-45   28
3.9.11   94
4.1   108
4.2   108
4.4   108
4.9   108

QUNITLILIAN, *Institutes of Oratory*
   5.9.14.   53

SAPPHO, Poem 58   58
SCRIBONIUS LARGUS, *Compositions of Drugs* 59   118-119
SENECA (ELDER)
   *Controversies*
   2.2.12   135
   7.3.4   128
SENECA (YOUNGER)
   *Epistles*
   56   9
   122.7-8   53
   *On Benefits*, 7.9   5
   *To Helvia, on Consolation*, 6   5
SILIUS ITALICUS, *Punica*,
   8.495-497   56
SUETONIUS
   *Augustus*, 79.2   117
   *Caesar*
   43   49
   49.4   71
   *Tiberius*, 43.2   40 n.35

TACITUS
   *Annals*
   1.54   50
   12.67   128
   *History*, 2.95   50
THEOCRITUS
   *Idyll*
   2.48-49   56
   17   30
THEOPHRASTUS
   *Enquiry into Plants*
   4.2   26
   9.2   78
   9.7   9
   9.9   67

9.11   67
9.19   67
*On Odours*, 13   116
*On Stones*   52
TIBULLUS
   1.5   55
   1.8.9–10   29, 30
   1.8.9–16   29
   1.8.17–26   29
   1.8.41–46   29
   2.5   108
   2.6   55

VALERIUS FLACCUS, *Argonautica*
      8.17   128
VARRO
   *De Lingua Latina*, 5.29.129   10
   *De Res Rusticae*, 1.2.3–7   26
VIRGIL
   *Aeneid*
      1.1   30

   3.216–218   128
   8.347–348   108
   8.354   127
   8.435   127
   *Eclogues*, 2.51–52   115
   *Georgics*
      1.56–57   26
      2.35–37   25
      2.56–59   26
      2.109–135   26
      2.126–130   39 n.27
      2.129   39 n.27
      2.136–176   26
      3.280–283   56
      3.282–283   39 n.27
      4.119   78
VITRUVIUS, *On Architecture*,
      8.6   69

XENOPHON, *Oeconomicus*,
      10.2–9   4

# General Index

abortifacients 32
accessorization 109–110 *see also*
    jewellery
acne 76, 77
Adonis 76, 131, 132
Agrippina the Elder 111
Ajax 102, 108
Alcyone 74
*alcyonea* 8, 71–74, 142
Alexandrians 2, 22, 25–26, 30,
    106, 116, 133
Alexis 2, 35
*aluta* 1–2, 100, 120
Amaryllis 104, 115
*amator*, Ovid as 28, 31, 86–87, 107
ammonium carbonate 64, 74, 118
ammonium chloride (Ammoniac salt)
    64, 77, 78, 80
*Amor / amor* 6, 19, 22–23, 28, 31, 33, 35,
    55, 58, 60, 125, 126
*Amores see* OVID (Passages index)
Andromache 97, 102, 108
Andromeda 116
Antoninus Liberalis 38 n.25
Aphrodite *see* Venus
Apollo 22, 84, 85, 87, 94, 108, 111
Aratus 25, 38 n.25, 39 n.26
Archigenes 8
Archilochus 34
Ariadne 93, 112, 139
Aristotle 56, 72
*ars* x, 4, 15–18, 37, 108, 112, 120, 121–122,
    134
*Ars Amatoria see* OVID (Passages
    index)
astringent 65, 78, 121
Athenaeus 2, 33
audiences, Ovid's 19–22, 28, 31–32, 48, 53,
    126, 135
Augustus 18–22, 33, 37 n.15, 94, 117, 120
Aurora 87, 115

Bacchant 92–93
Bacchus 93, 94, 98, 103, 107, 112, 139
bad breath 116, 118
baldness 10, 87, 89, 94–95, 110, 113
barley 46–47, 60–61, 62, 77, 78, 80, 119,
    138, 142
baths (bathing) 9, 18, 36 n.6, 36 n.7
beans 46, 67–68, 142
Berenice 30, 96
bitter vetch 60–61, 63, 64, 67, 88, 142
blemishes, hiding 2, 5, 48, 64, 73, 80, 120,
    138
blond hair 87–88
body odour 116, 133
Bona Dea 106, 124
Briseis 104, 116

*calamistrum* 93–94, 112, 133
Callimachus
    and *Amores* 30, 38 n.24, 39 n.29, 39
        n.31
    metaphrastics 25
    and Ovid 25
*candida* 59–60
*capilli see* hair
Catullus
    and *Amores* 30, 39 n.31, 40 n.32
    and Ovid 23
cedar 89–90, 92
Celsus 1, 61, 64, 65, 67, 68, 70, 76, 78
Ceres 44, 48, 87
*cerussa see* chalk
chalk 64, 68, 80, 104, 119
Chinese cloth 89
Cicero 53
    and *Remedia* 133–135
Circe 56
Claudian 120
clay 119
cleansers 64, 67, 68, 70, 73, 76–77, 78, 80,
    141, 142

## General Index

Cleopatra, *Kosmētikon* 8, 113
clothing 16, 20, 49, 51, 109–110, 113–116, 133
comb 10, 13, 14, 15, 91, 93, 110, 112, 122
*comes see* hair
corals 74
Corinna
   abortion 38 n.21, 75, 128
   baldness of 10, 30–31, 87, 90, 94–96
   beauty 55, 60
   *candida* 60
   hair of 89–90, 92–93, 94–96, 128
   and Ovid 19, 28, 86–87
cosmeceuticals 8–9, 11, 17, 35 n.1, 36 n.3, 55, 64, 74, 119
*creta see* chalk
*crines see* hair
Criton 8
'crocodile' dung 35, 80–81
crocus 115
*cultus*
   in *Amores* 88, 90, 92
   in *Ars Amatoria* 106–113, 119, 121, 124, 132–135
   in *Medicamina* 47–50, 51, 52, 53, 54–55, 57
   Ovid on (generally) x, 13, 15–18, 19–20, 25–27, 37 n, 37 n.11, 47
   Propertius on 29–30
   in *Remedia Amoris* 33–34, 37 n.11, 37 n.13, 47, 126–127
   Tibullus on 29
   Virgil on 26–27
Cupid 19, 27, 60
*cura* 25, 48
curling iron *see calamistrum*
Cybele 132, 133
Cypassis 19, 92

dating of Ovid's work xiii, 15, 22, 27, 38 n.18
*deliciae* 49–50
dentifrice 117–119
deodorant 9, 116
depilation 18, 72, 73, 117, 133
Diana 57, 111
didactic poetry 15–16, 19, 21, 22, 23–25, 26, 28, 32–33, 37 n.13, 39 n.29, 47, 106, 113, 126, 129

Dione *see* Venus
Dioscorides 9, 56, 65, 68, 69, 70, 72–74, 74, 76, 77, 78, 118, 123
*discriminale* 110
dung 9, 78, 80
dye (fabric) 49, 114–115
dye (hair) 7, 8, 12, 29, 49, 78, 87–88, 95–96, 110, 112–113, 128

Edwin Smith Papyrus 35 n.1
egg 60, 64, 118, 142
Elegy 22–23, 28
Elephantis 32, 40 n.35
emollients 64, 65–66, 76, 78, 141, 142
emulsifiers 64, 65, 67, 70, 77, 141, 142
epilation 117
*Epistles see* OVID (Passages index)
erodents 65, 70, 76–77
erotic handbooks/sex manuals 22, 32, 40 n.35
*exclusus amator* 28
exfoliants 9, 70, 77, 80, 141
exile poetry, Ovid's 37 n.14, 58–59
eyebrow-liner 120–121
eyebrows 3, 8, 120–121
eyeliner 120–121

*facies* 5, 48, 58
fading beauty 57–59
*faex* 80, 122
*Fasti see* OVID (Passages index)
fennel 47, 77–79, 142
Fonseca Bust 12, 112
*forma* 48, 52, 54–55, 58, 107, 110, 123, 134
foundation 4, 35, 69–70, 119, 120
frankincense 47, 65, 75–78, 80, 142
freckles 65, 70, 72

Galen 8, 32, 64, 72, 78, 81, 113
gems 26, 51–52, 94, 102
gold 51, 109–110, 114, 123–124
*Greek Magical Papyri* 81
*Greek Medical Papyri* 74
gum 60, 65, 75, 76, 91, 142

hair *see also* blond hair 8, 10, 12, 49, 51, 53, 87–88, 89–96, 110–113, 124, 133
hairdressers 19, 91, 92, 124
   Cypassis 19, 92

hair loss *see* baldness
hairpiece 12, 95
hairpieces *see also* wigs 12, 95
hair pin 10, 110
halitosis *see* bad breath
Harpies 128–129
hartshorn 60, 64, 80, 118
Hector 108
Heraclides 8
Hercules 112, 113, 139
*Heroides see* OVID (Passages index)
hind marrow 105, 123
Hippocrates (Hippocratic Corpus) 8–9, 72
*hippomanes* 39 n.27, 56
Hipponax 34
homeopathy 64–65, 68
homosexuality 29, 71, 133
honey 60, 61, 65, 67, 70, 71–72, 75, 77, 119, 142
Horace
   cosmetics 6, 65
   magic 55, 56
   misogyny 34–35, 58
   satire 35
   witches 55–57
hygiene, personal 116–119

*impudicitia* 7
incense 26, 74–75, 121
infusions 75, 77, 141
*ingenium* 57
iris 67–68, 70, 116
Isidorus
   *calamistrum* 93
   *discriminale* 110
ivory 14, 26, 49, 109

jewellery 5–6, 10, 12, 16–17, 36 n.3, 52, 109–110, 127
Julia Domna 111
Juvenal
   cosmetics 6, 7–8
   hairdressers 92

kaolinite 119
Kassel Apollo 111
kohl 120
*kommētikon* 8
*kosmētikon* 8

lanolin 7, 67, 122, 129
Laodamia 98, 102, 110
lead 4, 36 n.2, 67–69, 70, 80, 95, 142
*lena* 22, 37 n.11, 55
*lex Iulia* 18–22
*libertinae* 37 n.16, 106
Livia Drusilla 37 n.15, 111
Luna 57
lupin 61, 67–68, 69, 70, 72, 142
*luxuria* 16, 27

magic 29, 34, 55–57, 64–65, 68, 94–95, 112, 118, 128
marble 26, 60, 65, 109
*maritus* 53, 87
marrow 8, 123
Martial
   *aluta* 120
   cosmetics 6, 70
   hair 95, 113, 117
   hairdressers 92
mascara 65, 121
*matronae* 10, 17, 20–21
Medea 56, 128
*Medicamina see* OVID (Passages index)
medicine 32, 55, 65, 68, 75, 119, 123
men
   in *Ars Amatoria* 31, 132–135
   bathing 9, 36 n.7
   *cultus* 17–18, 53, 53–54, 132–135
   depilation 18, 117
   financial burden of women's adornment 7
   hair 8–9, 133
   hairdye 12, 112–113
   kept away from women's *cultus* 124
   modern men 1
   pounding 70–71
   *probitas* 58
   and purple 49
   in *Remedia Amoris* 33, 126
   women aiming to attract 107, 110
*meretrices* 7, 17, 20, 28, 87, 106
*Metamorphoses see* OVID (Passages index)
*militia amoris* 28
Mimnermus 58
mirror 10, 14, 58, 67, 110, 122
misogyny 34, 35

*mollitia* x, 17–18, 53
monobrow 120
moon 57
mortar and pestle 65
*mos* (*mores*) 57, 109
*munditia* 15, 16–18, 36 n.10, 119, 126, 133–134
*mundus muliebris* x, 10
*murex* 49, 80, 114, 115
Myron 17, 105, 123
myrrh 47, 65, 75, 76–77, 118, 142
Myrrha 76
myrtle 3, 4, 115
Mysia 116

narcissus 60–61, 65, 66, 70, 142
natron 67, 68, 70, 75–76, 113, 118, 142
Nicander, and Ovid 21, 24, 25, 38 n.25, 78
*nodus* 111

Octavia the Younger 111, 119
old age 29, 57–58
orris root 70

Parthians 124
patches 1–2, 120
peacock 54–55, 137
pearl-barley 61
pearls 5, 6, 52, 109
perfume 4, 6, 9, 18, 36 n.6, 70, 78, 141
Phaedra 131, 132
Pheidias 111
Philaenis 32
Phineus 126, 128, 129
*pietas* 59
pimples 61, 64, 65, 76, 77
plastic surgery
    ancient 1, 35 n.1
    modern 1, 4
poisonous substances 25, 56, 68, 80, 94, 95, 119, 128
Pompeii 9, 32, 93
poppy 61, 67, 80–81
potions 39 n.27, 56, 95, 128
*praeceptor amoris* 24, 29, 47, 124, 126
*praeceptor cultus* 47
*probitas* 58–59
Propertius
    cosmetics 6–7, 30

*cultus* 29, 93
*exclusus amator* 28
*militia amoris* 28
    and Ovid 22, 28, 29–30, 108
    Sabines 50
*servitium amoris* 28
    witchcraft 55
prostitutes *see also meretrices* 2–4, 35, 37 n.16, 87
*pudicitia* 7, 10, 96
*pudor* 20, 120
*puellae*
    in *Ars Amatoria* 31, 108, 116, 121, 124, 133
    in elegiac poetry generally 17, 28–29
    in *Medicamina* 48, 51–52, 57, 59–60
    in *Remedia Amoris* 33–35, 127–128
purple 49, 115
Pygmalion 123
*pyxis* (*pxyides*) 9–10, 13, 120, 122, 127, 129

recipes 59–81, 142
rings 49, 51–52, 122
rock salt 80
Rome
    empire 26, 27, 108–109
    trade x, 19, 75
roses
    oil 78
    petals 77, 78, 80, 120
rouge 4, 8, 35, 80–81, 119–120, 122

Sabine women 44, 50, 52, 107, 112
saffron 26, 104, 115, 120
salt 73, 78–79, 80, 119, 141, 142
*sapo* 88, 95
scent *see* perfume
Semonides 34
*servitium amoris* 28
sex manuals/erotic handbooks 22, 32, 40 n.35
Sextius Niger 74
shampoo 64, 65
silk 5, 53, 89
*sinus* 111
slaves 2, 37 n.16, 70, 92, 120
snakes 56, 78
soap 9, 65

spatulas 10, 36 n.6, 122
spelt 65, 66
spider's web 89
*splenium* 120 *see also aluta*
*stola* 20, 87
Sushruta Samhita 35 n.1
sweat 5, 116, 141

*tabellae* 32
Tatius 44, 50, 102, 107, 108
tattoos 2
Tecmessa 108
teeth 3, 4, 9, 73, 116–119, 123, 140 *see also* dentifrice
*tenera* 51, 60
Theseus 112, 132
Tibullus
    cosmetics 30
    *cultus* 29, 108
    *exclusus amator* 28
    *militia amoris* 28
    and Ovid 22, 28, 29, 30
    *servitium amoris* 28
    witchcraft 55
toga 20, 53, 132
*tractatrix* 92
*Triticum spelta* 65, 66
*tunica* 87
Tuscan seed 46, 60, 65, 142
Tyre 49

*unctrix* 92
un-Roman activities 19
*uxor* 87

*venena* 95, 128
Venus 9, 10, 20, 21, 48, 94, 105, 138
Venus Anadyomene 94, 123
vetch, bitter 46, 60–61, 63, 64, 67, 88, 142
Villa of the Mysteries 38 n.20
Virgil
    and *Amores* 30
    and *Medicamina* 23, 25–27
    and *Remedia Amoris* 33, 128
*virtus* 59
*vittae* 20, 37 n.15
*vultus* 23, 57, 67, 80

wheat 61, 65–66
wigs 12, 90, 95–96, 110, 112–113, 120, 124
witch/witchcraft 55–57, 94–95, 128
wives *see also matronae*
    adulturous wives 7, 18
    Berenice 96
    Corinna 87
    and *cultus* 53
    *nupta* 53, 59
    Ovid's wife 58–59
    *probitas* 58, 59
    *uxor* 87
    wifely virtues 50, 96
wool 21, 105, 122
wool grease *see* lanolin
wrinkles 45, 46, 48, 57, 58, 64, 75, 77

www.ingramcontent.com/pod-product-compliance
Lightning Source LLC
Chambersburg PA
CBHW050140240426
43673CB00043B/1736